THE DEFENDING ARMY

JOURNEY THROUGH THE MIND AND BODY

TIME® LIFE BOOKS

Other Publications:
WEIGHT WATCHERS® SMART CHOICE RECIPE COLLECTION
TRUE CRIME
THE AMERICAN INDIANS
THE ART OF WOODWORKING
LOST CIVILIZATIONS
ECHOES OF GLORY
THE NEW FACE OF WAR
HOW THINGS WORK
WINGS OF WAR
CREATIVE EVERYDAY COOKING
COLLECTOR'S LIBRARY OF THE UNKNOWN
CLASSICS OF WORLD WAR II
TIME-LIFE LIBRARY OF CURIOUS AND UNUSUAL FACTS
AMERICAN COUNTRY
VOYAGE THROUGH THE UNIVERSE
THE THIRD REICH
THE TIME-LIFE GARDENER'S GUIDE
MYSTERIES OF THE UNKNOWN
TIME FRAME
FIX IT YOURSELF
FITNESS, HEALTH & NUTRITION
SUCCESSFUL PARENTING
HEALTHY HOME COOKING
UNDERSTANDING COMPUTERS
LIBRARY OF NATIONS
THE ENCHANTED WORLD
THE KODAK LIBRARY OF CREATIVE PHOTOGRAPHY
GREAT MEALS IN MINUTES
THE CIVIL WAR
PLANET EARTH
COLLECTOR'S LIBRARY OF THE CIVIL WAR
THE EPIC OF FLIGHT
THE GOOD COOK
WORLD WAR II
HOME REPAIR AND IMPROVEMENT
THE OLD WEST

For information on and a full description of any of the
Time-Life Books series listed above, please call
1-800-621-7026 or write:
Reader Information
Time-Life Customer Service
P.O. Box C-32068
Richmond, Virginia 23261-2068

THE DEFENDING ARMY

JOURNEY THROUGH THE MIND AND BODY

BY THE EDITORS OF TIME-LIFE BOOKS
ALEXANDRIA, VIRGINIA

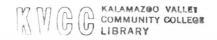

CONSULTANTS:

PAUL J. COTE teaches at Georgetown University's Division of Molecular Virology and Immunology, Rockville, Maryland. His special research interest is the immunology of hepatitis B virus.

NICHOLAS HALL, a professor of psychoimmunology in the Department of Psychiatry, University of South Florida, Tampa, counsels patients to fight cancer actively with visual imagery. His research examines mechanisms of how the brain and the immune system communicate.

HOWARD M. JOHNSON teaches in the Department of Microbiology and Cell Science, University of Florida, Gainesville. He is a consultant in sickle cell anemia to the National Heart, Lung and Blood Institute in Bethesda, Maryland.

PHYLLIS KIND is a cellular immunologist at the George Washington University Medical Center, Washington, D.C. Her major scientific interest is the regulation of the immune response; most recently she has been studying the interaction of macrophages and T cells.

JOHN R. ORTALDO, chief of the Laboratory of Experimental Immunology at the National Cancer Institute, Frederick, Maryland, focuses his research on immunology against tumors at the cellular level.

TERENCE PHILLIPS is director of the immunochemistry laboratories at George Washington University, Washington, D.C. His research interests include mechanisms of immune regulation and the analysis of antigen structure and function.

NOEL R. ROSE has done extensive research on autoimmune diseases, especially those of the thyroid; his research involves both human beings and experimental animals. He teaches in the Department of Immunology at the Johns Hopkins School of Hygiene and Public Health, Baltimore.

ARTHUR M. SILVERSTEIN wrote A *History of Immunology*, published in 1989. Retired from teaching, he continues his studies at the Institute of the History of Medicine, the Johns Hopkins University, Baltimore.

BARBARA A. TORRES teaches in the Department of Microbiology and Cell Science, University of Florida, Gainesville. She is engaged in research on antigens and superantigens.

JOURNEY THROUGH THE MIND AND BODY

TIME-LIFE BOOKS

EDITOR-IN-CHIEF: John L. Papanek

Executive Editor: Roberta Conlan
Director of Editorial Resources:
  Elise D. Ritter-Clough
Executive Art Director: Ellen Robling
Director of Photography and Research:
  John Conrad Weiser
Editorial Board: Russell B. Adams, Jr.,
  Dale M. Brown, Janet Cave, Robert
  Doyle, Jim Hicks, Rita Thievon Mullin,
  Robert Somerville, Henry Woodhead
Assistant Director of Editorial Resources:
  Norma E. Shaw

PRESIDENT: John D. Hall

Vice President, Director of Marketing:
  Nancy K. Jones
Vice President, New Product Development:
  Neil Kagan
Director of Production Services: Robert N. Carr
Production Manager: Marlene Zack
Director of Technology: Eileen Bradley
Supervisor of Quality Control: James King

Editorial Operations

Production: Celia Beattie
Library: Louise D. Forstall
Computer Composition: Deborah G. Tait
  (Manager), Monika D. Thayer, Janet
  Barnes Syring, Lillian Daniels
Interactive Media Specialist: Patti H. Cass

Time-Life Books is a division of
  Time Life Inc.

PRESIDENT AND CEO: John M. Fahey, Jr.

SERIES EDITOR: Robert Somerville
Administrative Editor: Judith W. Shanks

Editorial Staff for The Defending Army
Art Directors: Rebecca Mowrey, Barbara
  Sheppard, Fatima Taylor
Picture Editors: Charlotte Marine Fullerton,
  Kristin Baker Hanneman
Text Editors: Lee Hassig, Jim Watson
Associate Editor/Research: Ruth Goldberg
Assistant Editor/Research: M. Kevan Miller
Writer: Mark Galan
Assistant Art Director: Sue Pratt
Copyeditor: Donna D. Carey
Editorial Assistant: Julia Kendrick
Picture Coordinators: Mark C. Burnett,
  Paige Henke

Special Contributors:
George Constable, Tucker Coombe,
Marge duMond, Juli Duncan, Laura Foreman, Betsy Hanson, Doug Harbrecht,
Marilyn Johnson, Barbara Mallen, Eliot
Marshall, Brian Miller, Diana Loercher
Pazicky, Peter Pocock, Elizabeth J. Sherman, Linda Smith, Elizabeth Winters
(text); Susan Blair, Gretchen Case, Craig
Chapin, Elaine Friebele, Anna Gedrich,
Stephanie Summers Henke, Gevene
Hertz, Jocelyn Lindsay, Nathalie op de
Beeck (research); Barbara L. Klein (overread and index); John Drummond (design); Heidi Fritschel (copy).

Correspondents:
Elisabeth Kraemer-Singh (Bonn); Otto
Gibius, Robert Kroon (Geneva); Christine
Hinze (London); Christina Lieberman
(New York); Maria Vincenza Aloisi (Paris);
Mary Johnson (Stockholm); Ann Natanson
(Rome); Dick Berry (Tokyo). Valuable assistance was also provided by Elizabeth
Brown (New York).

**Library of Congress
Cataloging-in-Publication Data**

The Defending army / by the editors of
Time-Life Books.
  p. cm. — (Journey through the mind
and body)
  Includes bibliographical references and
index.
  ISBN 0-7835-1012-8 (v. 4 : trade)
  ISBN 0-7835-1013-6 (v. 4 : library)
  1. Immunity—Popular works.
2. Immune system—Popular works.
I. Time-Life Books. II. Series.
QR181.7.D44 1994
616.07'9—dc20   93-33512

This volume is one of a series that
explores the fascinating inner universe
of the human mind and body.

CONTENTS

1————————————

2————————————

3————————————

4————————————

8 **DRAWING THE BATTLE LINES**

31 Equipped for the Struggle

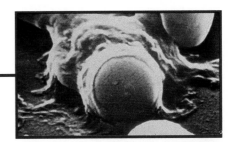

38 **AN EDUCATED DEFENSE**

61 The Call to Arms

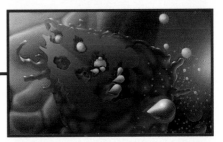

70 **IMMUNITY OUT OF BALANCE**

94 Sensitive to a Fault

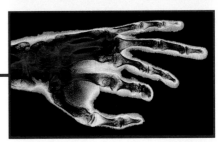

100 **THE HEALING POWERS OF MIND**

124 Detecting Renegades: The Immune System and Cancer

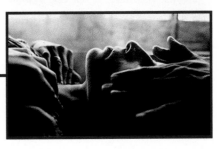

134 Glossary **136** Bibliography **139** Index **144** Acknowledgments **144** Picture Credits

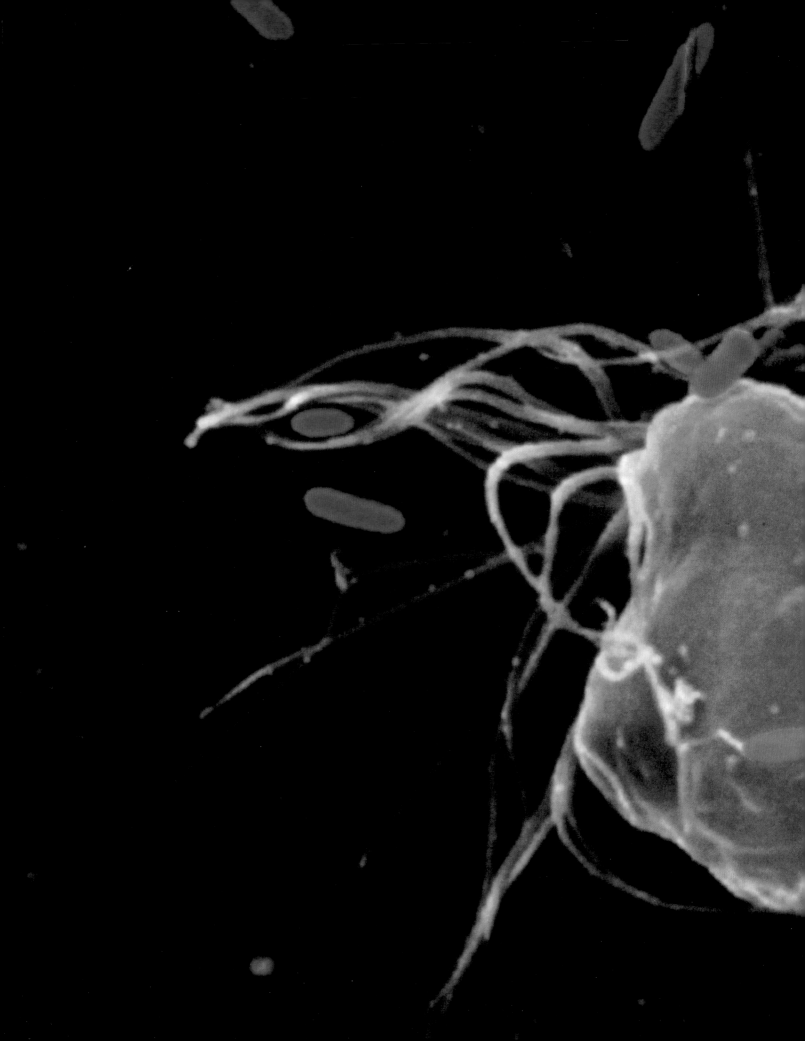

1

Drawing the Battle Lines

Witchcraft is not the sort of subject that ordinarily turns up in medical publications. Nevertheless, it did find its way into the venerable *Journal of the American Medical Association*, in the issue of May 15, 1981. A doctor named Richard Kirkpatrick of St. John's Hospital in Longview, Washington, told of a woman who had come to him with a debilitating disease known as lupus erythematosus. Kirkpatrick wrote to report his bafflement—not with the disease, which has well-defined symptoms, but with the only form of treatment that had worked. After Kirkpatrick's own efforts failed, the patient's lupus had apparently been cured by a witch doctor.

Kirkpatrick explained that the patient, "Lucy," who was 28 years old when he met her, had an unusual personal history. She grew up in a rural village in the Philippines, where she bore two children by a Filipino man. Lucy had never married, but after meeting a U.S. serviceman stationed in her country, she decided to become his wife. The American adopted her two children and moved the family to the United States. Soon afterward, Lucy grew weak and anemic. She suffered from swollen tissues, kidney malfunction, and fatigue. When she visited Kirkpatrick, the doctor recognized her symptoms. Lupus occurs when a person's immune sys-

PRECEDING PAGE: The immune system's primary scavenger, a macrophage *(yellow)* homes in on *E. coli* bacteria *(purple)*, ignoring nearby red blood cells. The ropelike extensions—called pseudopods—are cellular appendages that the macrophage uses to snag any foreign substance it encounters.

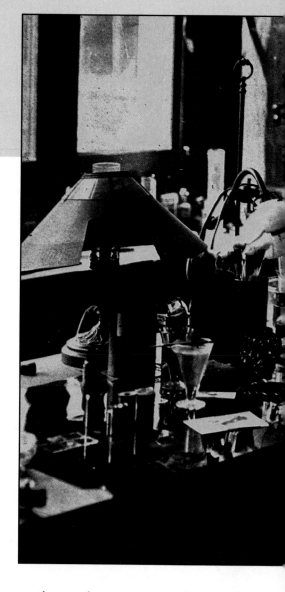

tem—the complex defensive apparatus whose job it is to fight invading organisms—gets confused and begins attacking the body's own blood and tissue. It can be fatal if left untreated.

Lucy tested positive for lupus, and Kirkpatrick prescribed prednisone, a drug that reduces inflammation. It seemed to help for a while, but the patient relapsed. When Kirkpatrick recommended a higher dose of prednisone, Lucy refused and soon thereafter left for her home village in the Philippines. Kirkpatrick knew that abruptly breaking off prednisone therapy was dangerous, and he worried that Lucy might come to harm. But three weeks later she returned. "Much to the surprise of distraught family members and skeptical physicians," Kirkpatrick reported, "she was 'normal.'" According to her own account, the illness had resulted from a hex put on her by the father of her children—and the cure had come about when a witch doctor lifted the curse. Back in the United States, she refused any further medication and was doing so well that she was later able to give birth to a healthy girl.

Kirkpatrick could not explain what had happened. He consulted other doctors but never heard a good medical analysis of the disease's remission. On the one hand, the witch doctor may have applied a treatment not known to traditional science. On the

other hand, conventional medicine might in fact have an explanation for Lucy's sudden improvement. It is well known that the immune system can be weakened by stress. Lucy's belief that she had been cursed, and her consequent fear, may have reduced the effectiveness of her immune system. The visit to the witch doctor, then, might have given her an emotional boost that found expression in her ability to rally against the lupus. Whatever their cause, the beneficial effects lasted only temporarily. In the end, the disease overpowered her, and she died several years later.

Lupus and other diseases that affect the immune system are particularly difficult to treat because the immune system is itself a very complicated matter. Immunity is not centered in one place, nor is it controlled by a single organ. It is an army with no commanding general—a panoply of chemicals and cells employing various strategies for dealing with a wide range of enemies. Some of the defenders take on any and every foe they meet, while others are designed to target specific adversaries. In ways still far from fully understood, these many components take cues from one

another, working in teams and responding moment by moment to changes in the body's internal environment.

In fact, only within the past 30 years have researchers begun to sort out details of how the elements of the immune system communicate with one another and divide up their tasks. Scientists have discovered an array of inspectors, identification monitors, messengers, and others all devoted to the single cause of defending a person's "self"—those components recognized by the immune

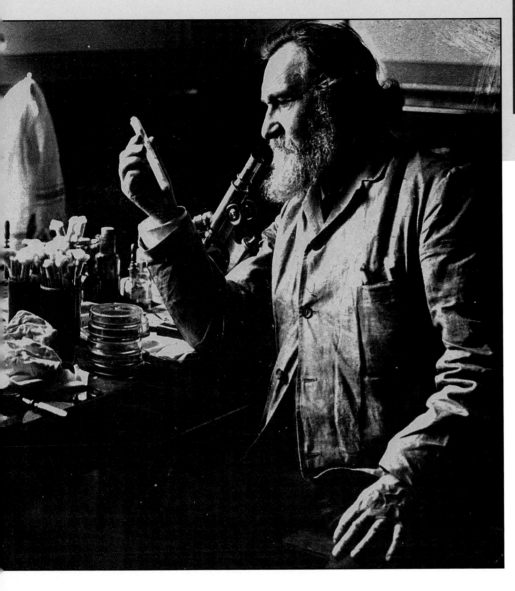

ber previous battles, so that they can mount a second attack in a hurry should an old enemy return.

Critical to all these functions is the tagging scheme, based on a person's unique genetic makeup, that labels cells in the body with a flag that says either "self" or "other." Only after alien or infected cells have been so marked can immune cells go about their duties of targeting and destroying them. Indeed, some of the most insidious diseases afflicting humans depend for their success on subverting this labeling mechanism—disguising other as self or, as in the case of lupus, causing the immune system to attack self as if it were other.

Understanding the nuances of how the immune system works is made all the more difficult by the microscopic scale of its players. Some immune cells measure only millionths of a meter in diameter, and a change in one molecule on their surface can profoundly affect the role they play. The enemy can be even smaller and just as mutable. Precisely because of these minuscule dimensions, for centuries no one even imagined that life-and-death battles between opposing legions of invaders and defenders were taking place within the body.

system as part of the individual that it belongs to and serves.

At the outermost boundary of the protected territory is the skin, the primary barrier against the threat of infection by bacteria and viruses. The body's largest organ, the skin is coated with defensive chemicals that deter hostile organisms. Should any penetrate this perimeter, however,

more defenders lie in wait. A bacterium that succeeds in reaching the bloodstream, for example, might meet a macrophage—a large cell whose job it is to devour intruders. A virus might be able to elude the powerful macrophages and hide for days within a cell. But sooner or later, it is likely to be marked as hostile by antibodies, proteins that patrol the bloodstream and help direct counterattacks. Along with scouts and soldiers, the body's protective army also includes platoons of cells designed to remember

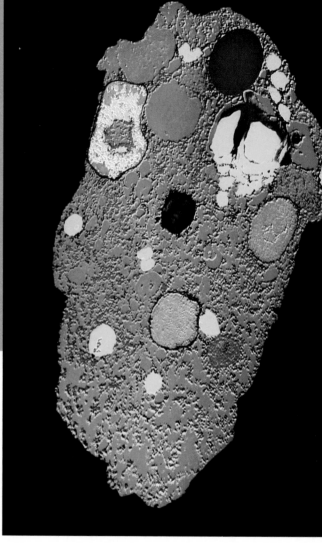

But in the 1600s, a Dutch amateur scientist set the stage for a revolution in awareness with an instrument that for the first time opened a window on the rich and varied microbial world.

Born to a family of brewers in 1632, Antoni van Leeuwenhoek grew up in middle-class comfort in the town of Delft. He went into business as a dry-goods merchant, but his real passion —his obsession, in fact—was studying the magnifying power of lenses. He began to grind his own, buying the equipment from a maker of eyeglass-es. Leeuwenhoek devoted all his free time to this pursuit, selecting glass, shaping it, polishing it, and crafting lenses that got finer and smaller as he progressed. He then began mount-ing his lenses on handmade metal structures for easier focusing—there-by fashioning the first microscopes, with which he examined everything from the parts of a fly to the structure of the hairs of beaver and elk.

Little is known of Leeuwenhoek's early work; for 20 years he shared his insight with no one but his own fami-ly. But word of his exotic interests got around Delft, and eventually a scholar named Reinier de Graaf paid a visit. Graaf was so impressed by Leeuwen-hoek's discoveries that he wrote to the recently formed Royal Society of London, the world's first scientific or-ganization, urging it to request a re-port directly from the microscope's

inventor. The society did write to Leeuwen-hoek in 1673, and he responded with a long and rather windy letter. Translated from Dutch, it was entitled: "A Spec-imen of some Obser-vations made by a Microscope contrived by Mr. Leeuwenhoek, concerning Mould upon the Skin, Flesh, etc.; the Sting of a Bee, etc." The Royal Society was in-trigued and asked Leeuwen-hoek to furnish more reports. Over the next few years, he inundated them with ram-bling epistles, almost every one of which contained at least a few descriptive gems.

One letter held particularly stirring news. It noted that on one occasion Leeuwenhoek had decided to focus his microscope on a sample of rainwater. To his amazement, he saw tiny creatures swimming within it, each one, he wrote, "a thousand times smaller than the eye of a louse." A later report on another type of sample noted that there are "more animals living . . . on

the teeth in a man's mouth than there are men in a whole kingdom."

The descriptions of these "wretched beasties," as Leeuwenhoek called them, left some members of the Roy-al Society skeptical. Nevertheless, the society asked to buy one of his pre-cious microscopes so that members might see the creatures for them-selves. Leeuwenhoek refused to sell, but his monopoly on the microscope did not last long: The society com-

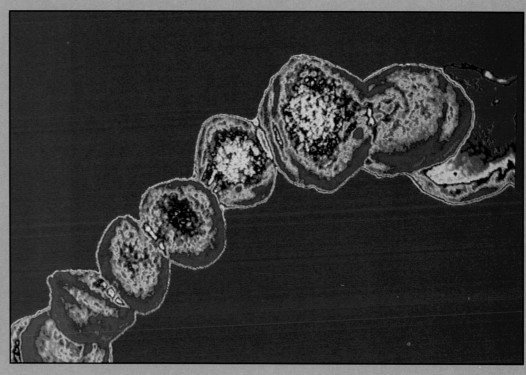

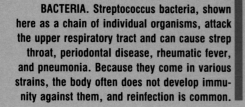

AMOEBA. Lurking in unclean food and water, this one-celled organism causes digestive-tract disorders, including some forms of dysentery. The one shown here has ingested red blood cells *(green)*. Internal bleeding can result from an amoeba's attack on cells in the intestinal walls and, in severe cases, the liver.

BACTERIA. Streptococcus bacteria, shown here as a chain of individual organisms, attack the upper respiratory tract and can cause strep throat, periodontal disease, rheumatic fever, and pneumonia. Because they come in various strains, the body often does not develop immunity against them, and reinfection is common.

missioned Robert Hooke—later a famous scientist in his own right—to build an instrument for the members. Hooke complied, and on November 15, 1677, he brought the new device to a society meeting. The incredulous members then saw what Leeuwenhoek had been telling them about. The discovery lifted the curtain on an entire new universe in miniature.

Still, it was by no means immediately apparent that Leeuwenhoek's "beasties" were the agents of illness. The popular notion then and for many years to come—known as the miasma theory of disease—was that sickness resulted from exposure to ill-defined noxious vapors, or "bad air." According to this view, the kinds of microorganisms observed by Leeuwenhoek and others were symptoms rather than causes of disease—a belief based in part on an unwillingness to accept that such tiny creatures could wreak such havoc on their human and animal hosts.

Some 200 years after Leeuwenhoek's discoveries, however, an alternative hypothesis—the germ theory of disease—eventually won out. Its main champion was the famed French chemist Louis Pasteur, whose first breakthrough was demonstrating that bacteria are responsible for the fermentation of beer and wine. Building on this evidence, Pasteur went on to confirm the findings of a German pathologist named Robert Koch, who had devised a series of experiments that appeared to show that various types of infectious disease could be traced to the action of microorganisms. By the late 1870s, the role of these infinitesimal beings in both the development and the spread of disease was firmly established.

The next great question, of course, was how the body goes about warding off infection and disease, which it clearly has the ability to do. For his part, Pasteur focused on the rather surprising discovery that the body can acquire immunity to specific diseases (*Chapter* 2), and as a result he was instrumental in developing new treatments to several devastating afflictions. As for the body's innate disease-fighting power, there were

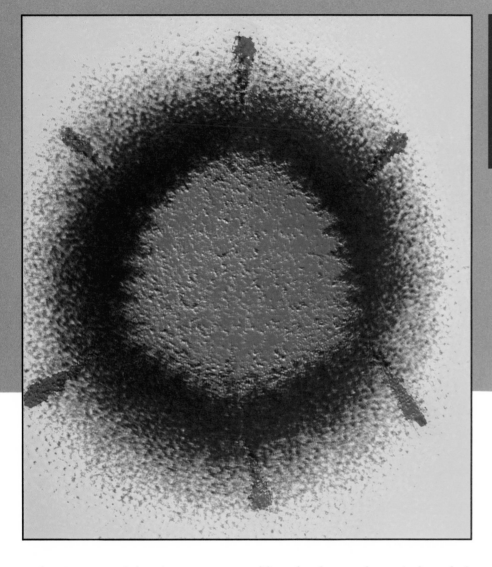

at the time several theories as to the mechanisms involved, but little evidence—until Élie Metchnikoff appeared on the scene claiming that certain cells in the body are expressly designed to fend off foreign assaults.

Metchnikoff, born in 1845 in Ivanovka on the Russian steppe, studied zoology at several of the great universities of Germany and Russia. A brilliant and volatile student, Metchnikoff led a tumultuous life as a young man. His first major project at the University of Giessen, an investigation of the

life cycle of a roundworm in frogs, led to a dispute: He made novel discoveries, only to learn that his professor had stolen his work and published it as his own. Metchnikoff left the university and moved to Naples, where he won a fellowship from a marine biological laboratory to study sponges. In a pattern typical of his life, he quarreled with a colleague—in this

case, over the nervous system of the sponge—and decamped. His next stop was St. Petersburg, where he nearly died of influenza. Although he recovered, the young woman who helped him through the sickness, and whom he married, soon died herself of tuberculosis. Despondent, Metchnikoff attempted suicide.

Fortunately for science, Metchnikoff miscalculated a self-administered dose of morphine and survived. In 1875, at age 30, he married again, this time to an adoring teenager named Olga Belokopitova. The newlyweds moved to Odessa, where Metchnikoff fell once more into despair, this time over the poor progress of his career. He injected himself with what he thought was a lethal dose of a fever-causing microorganism. But again, his suicide attempt failed. After a long

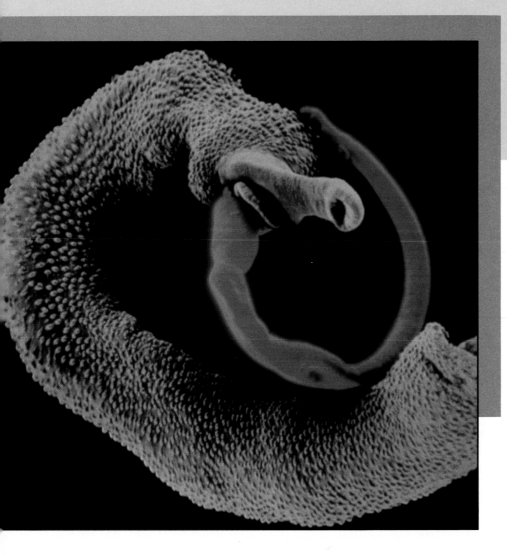

illness he recovered, and as he did, his fortunes began to improve.

With income inherited from Olga's parents in 1881, the Metchnikoffs moved to Messina, Italy, where the temperamental Russian began studying a subject that had always engaged his curiosity—the causes of inflammation in animal tissue. In this pursuit, he would make the most important discovery of his career. One day in 1883, he chose for inspection a star-fish larva, an excellent object of research because its transparent body allowed him to observe its insides without killing it. As he gazed at it, he had an inspiration: Cells within the body might serve as defenders against invasions of foreign material.

Metchnikoff went to his rose garden and plucked a thorn, poking it into the larva to see what defensive response would ensue. The next day he looked at the specimen and noticed that the thorn had indeed been surrounded by a swarm of cells. He concluded that his theory was correct and devoted the next 25 years to exploring the protective role of cells that he called phagocytes, from the Greek *phagos* (to eat) and *cyte* (cell).

Applying his theory to humans as well as to animals, Metchnikoff said that the white blood cells in pus are actually phagocytes that catch and digest invading particles. This assertion clashed with the prevailing opinion that pus was an undesirable substance, a transmitter of disease throughout the body. But as research proceeded, it became clear that Metchnikoff was right, and by 1886 he was known around the world for his work. He moved to Paris and established himself at the Pasteur Institute.

Metchnikoff identified two broad categories of phagocytes, but today these two families include many more subdivisions, reflecting the great variety of cell shapes and functions that have been discovered. For example, scientists now recognize two distinct types of the large white blood cells called macrophages. Some remain affixed to tissues and to blood vessel linings, particularly in the spleen and liver, ready to dispose of any foreign material that comes their way. Others circulate throughout the body seeking out invaders and zeroing in as needed on trouble spots, such as where

The First Line of Defense

The human body comes equipped with all sorts of sophisticated defenses, from roving scavengers and potent chemicals to special cells designed to "remember" the identity of a foe long after an initial attack. But among the most important protections are the physical barriers that help keep harmful agents from infiltrating the body in the first place.

The body's prime armor is the skin. Composed of multiple layers, it essentially provides a series of obstacles that stand in the way of potential invaders. Its shielding properties are augmented by hair, which brushes away foreign matter and microorganisms before they can even reach the skin's surface.

Certain interior parts of the body benefit from similar protection. For example, the respiratory and digestive tracts, which are exposed to the outside environment through the mouth and nose, are lined with an equivalent to the skin known as the mucous membrane. The sticky mucus it produces serves to trap foreign particles, which are then expelled through such actions as coughing or sneezing. In addition, some cells of the mucous membrane have thin, hairlike projections called cilia that help sweep out debris.

As detailed on the next two pages, these physical barriers employ a variety of techniques and work together with other defensive agents to keep most disease-causing microbes and threatening substances at bay.

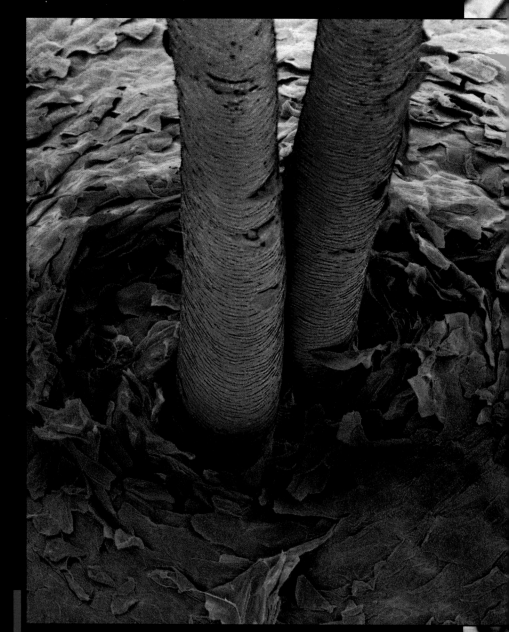

HAIR AND SKIN. Shown at 320 times their actual size, two hairs rise from a patchy field of skin on a human scalp. They are rooted in an underlying skin layer, in small cavities called follicles.

THE MUCOUS MEMBRANE. Magnified more than 4,000 times, tentacle-like cilia project above mucus-producing goblet cells in a human trachea. The waving action of the cilia moves mucus up and out of the respiratory tract at the rate of about one inch per hour.

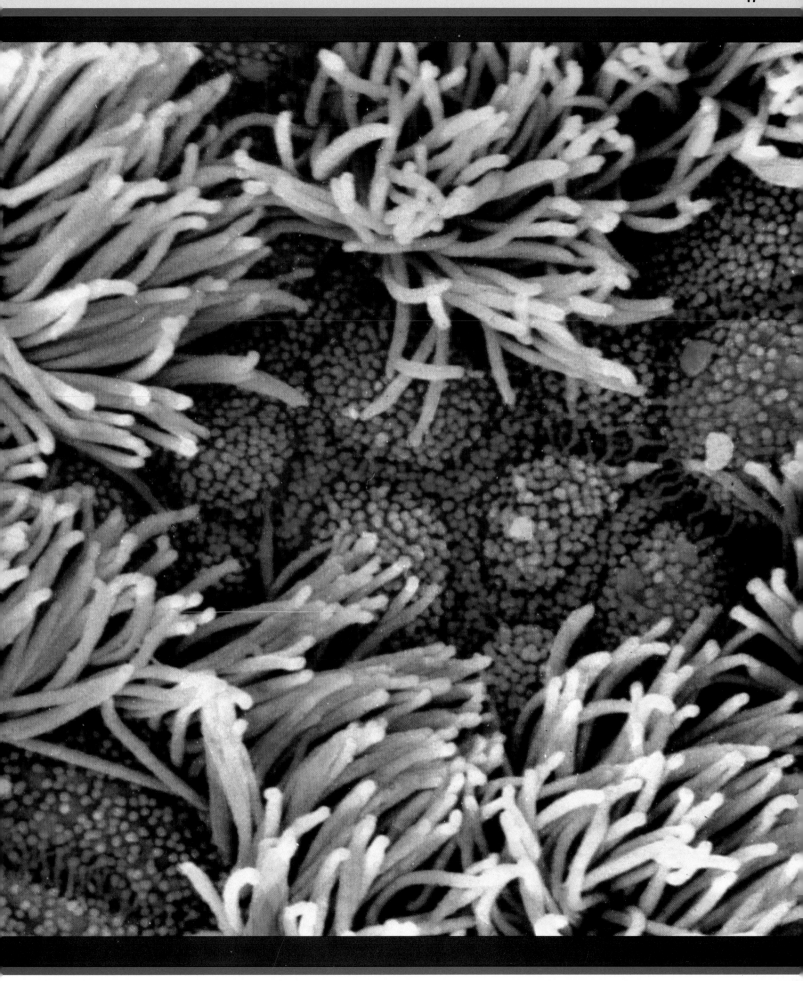

Dispatching the Enemy

Besides barring the way to invaders, the first line of defense typically ensures that pathogens are either removed or destroyed before they can do any harm. The skin, for example, is itself covered with a thin film consisting of various secretions, including sweat and oils, that constantly rinse off the surface and have antiseptic qualities as well. Other body fluids, such as tears and mucus, contain lysozyme, an immune system agent that breaks chemical bonds in the cell walls of bacteria, killing them.

Even so, some microbes do manage to penetrate the surface, but the cells there are so tightly bound together—by the same protein as in fingernails—that intruders usually get trapped; they are then carried away as the dead cells in this layer flake off.

Supplementing these defenses are the so-called friendly flora—foreign organisms that inhabit mucous membranes and are also found on the skin; they consume nutrients that otherwise would support more harmful germs. These microbes have, in effect, established a live-and-let-live relationship with the body.

SWEAT. Microscopic beads of sweat appear 200 times their actual size in this electron micrograph. As well as cooling the skin, sweat carries off harmful microorganisms and contains acidic chemicals that create a hostile environment for bacteria.

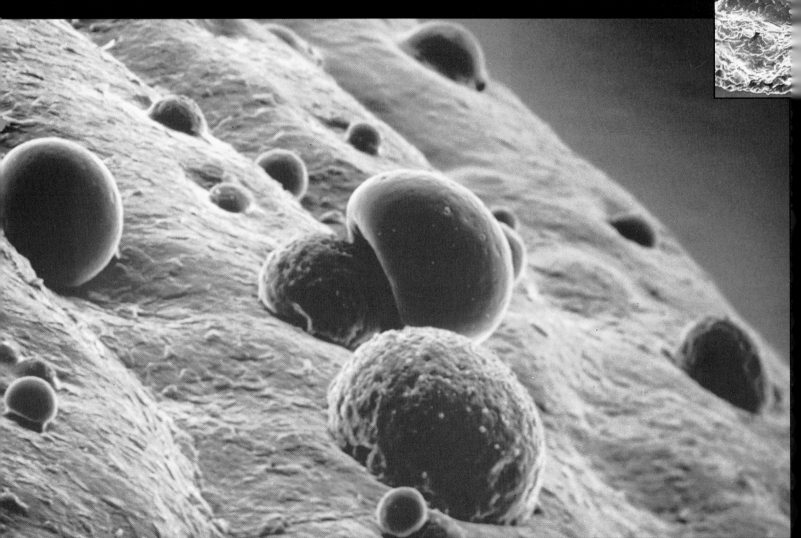

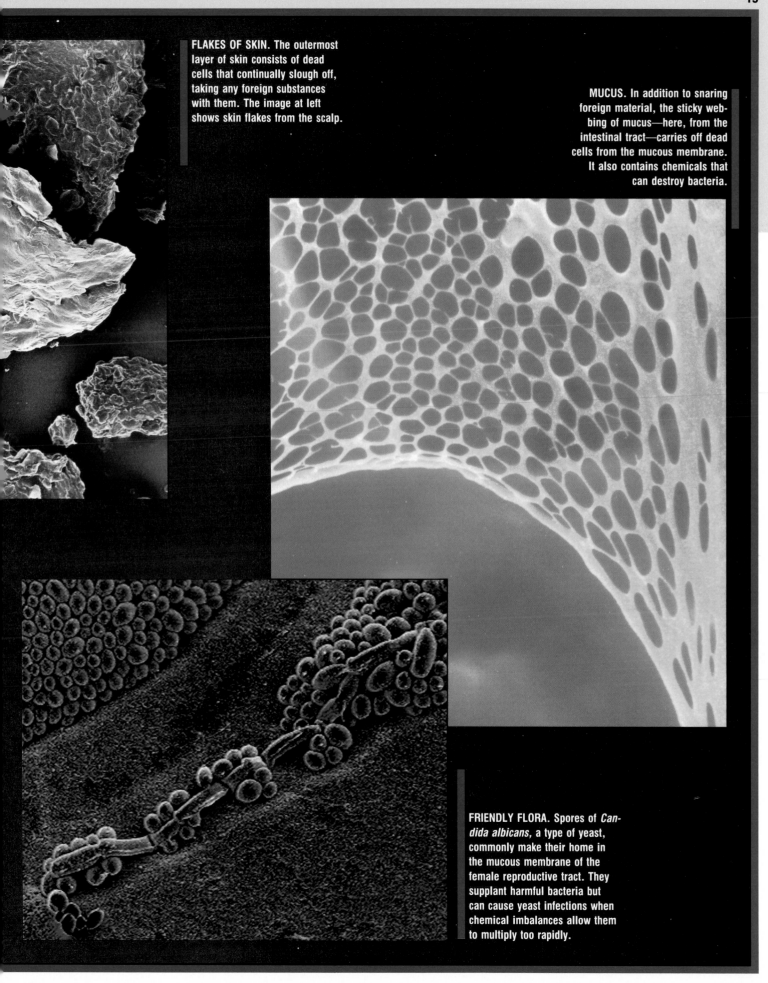

FLAKES OF SKIN. The outermost layer of skin consists of dead cells that continually slough off, taking any foreign substances with them. The image at left shows skin flakes from the scalp.

MUCUS. In addition to snaring foreign material, the sticky webbing of mucus—here, from the intestinal tract—carries off dead cells from the mucous membrane. It also contains chemicals that can destroy bacteria.

FRIENDLY FLORA. Spores of *Candida albicans*, a type of yeast, commonly make their home in the mucous membrane of the female reproductive tract. They supplant harmful bacteria but can cause yeast infections when chemical imbalances allow them to multiply too rapidly.

tissue has been damaged. It is also known today that phagocytes contribute to the destruction of invaders in ways other than by ingesting them directly. In elaborate interactions that Metchnikoff could scarcely have imagined, chemicals secreted by phagocytes help to regulate all the body's immune responses, from the clotting of blood to triggering the release of various hormones that fight infection (*pages* 61-69).

Vital as they are, phagocytes, produced in bone marrow, are by no means the only cells involved in defending the body. Just as essential is another family of cells called lymphocytes, which also arise in bone marrow but undergo further development in various organs of the lymphatic system such as the thymus, spleen, lymph nodes, and tonsils. Lymphocytes assume a number of roles, one of the most important of which is acting as command-and-control relay points for regulating a series of defensive responses by other substances. Unlike phagocytes, which try to kill any alien material they encounter, lymphocytes have to identify an enemy before they can attack it. Lymphocytes are the immune system's specialists, programmed to recognize specific types of antigens, the name given to all invading molecules capable of triggering an immune response.

Although knowledge of the multi-form complexities of immune function was many years in the future, it was Metchnikoff who, in discovering phagocytes, laid the groundwork for all the studies on cellular immunity that followed. He received the Nobel Prize in 1908 for his efforts, but fame may have hardened him in his views. In his later years Metchnikoff began insisting that all forms of immunity derived from phagocytes. Even as it became evident at the turn of the century that there was some other material in the bloodstream that helped support the body's defense system, he refused to yield ground. He declared that other blood-based, or "humoral," immune factors—if any existed—were merely by-products of his favorite family of cells. A heated debate ensued between defenders of cellular and humoral theories. But the truth, as so often is the case in science, is that both were partly right.

In the last years of the 19th century, several researchers working independently helped to establish that there was more to the immune system than phagocytes. One of the first to uncover such evidence was American biologist George Nuttall, who began attending the prestigious University of Göttingen in 1886 to write a dissertation in microbiology. While there, he learned of a new theory that his colleagues had proposed, claiming that blood serum—that is, the clear fluid part of blood, separate from red and white blood cells and clotting proteins—could kill bacteria.

To test this notion, Nuttall injected a sample of the bacteria that cause anthrax—a deadly and highly contagious affliction primarily affecting cattle and sheep—into frogs, and he observed as phagocytes rushed to mount a defense. Indeed, the phagocytes did devour some of the anthrax bacteria. But, Nuttall noted, many of the invading organisms appeared to be killed in the "empty" zone where no phagocytes were at work; blood serum alone was somehow destroying them. Obviously something other than cells was doing the work, although Nuttall could not say what that something might be. Based on observations such as these, Nuttall and his allies waged an intense intellectual battle against the cellular school, arguing that there had to be another substance involved in the immune response.

A major contributor to the debate was a German bacteriologist named Emil von Behring, who had become interested in the subject of immunity not long after Pasteur first demonstrated the role of microorganisms in

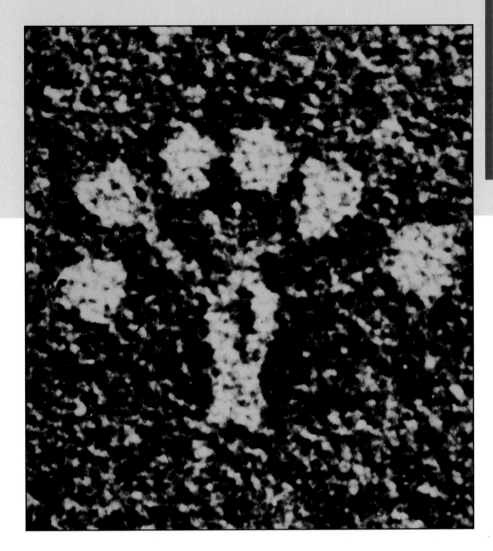

The protein molecule at left starts the chain reaction known as the complement cascade, in which about 20 related proteins normally inactive in the blood come to the aid of antibodies. When an invading antigen attaches to a cell and an antibody in turn binds to the antigen, this molecule reacts by binding to the stem of the Y-shaped antibody, and the chemical cascade begins. One of its results is the puncturing of the affected cell's walls and the destruction of the antigen.

disease. Early in the 1880s, Behring had experimented with administering wound-cleansing disinfectants internally to see if they would kill disease organisms in test animals. Not surprisingly, the results were poor: The toxic chemicals proved more effective at killing the animals than did the diseases themselves.

But Behring continued to experiment, and several years later a different approach yielded interesting results. In 1890 he discovered that an immunized animal's blood serum by itself, with no phagocytes present,

could counteract disease. Further research showed that the serum provided immunity by working against toxins that had been released by the disease organisms; as a result, Behring called the unknown substance in the serum antitoxin. In any event, he had succeeded in proving that a cellular defense was not the only factor at work in the immune system.

In the years immediately following, other researchers helped fill in the picture about the exact nature of Behring's antitoxin. By the middle of the 1890s, Belgian bacteriologist Jules Bordet had figured out that two components were working in tandem in this version of the immune response. One was a class of protein mole-

cules—already identified by Behring himself and another colleague and later dubbed antibodies—that were very specifically attuned to particular types of antigens; a given antibody appeared only in blood serum from an animal immunized to the corresponding disease. The other component was a more complex protein compound that was found to be present in any sample of blood serum, whether or not an immunity had developed within it. In simple terms, Bordet discovered that humoral immunity involved first an antigen-specific reaction by antibodies, and then follow-up destructive action by this more generic second component, which became known as complement because of its complementary role in the immune response.

Further details regarding humoral immunity led to important new breakthroughs in understanding the mechanisms of acquired immunity and just how the immune system gears itself to specific types of invaders. But there was much still to learn about the overall workings of the body's defenses. For instance, phagocytes, antibodies, and the complement proteins all operate only within the body, transported by the blood and lymphatic vessels. During the 1920s, however, scientists discovered a general family of immune system chemicals that also defend more exposed sectors. They are abundant in tears and nasal mucus, on the lining of the throat, and in sputum. The man who identified them, Scottish bacteriologist Alexander Fleming, later became famous as the discoverer of penicillin. But for many years, his early and important research on this innate bactericide—known as lysozyme (from Greek roots roughly meaning "enzyme that destroys or breaks down") —was largely unrecognized.

Fleming made the discovery, according to his lab assistant and colleague V. D. Allison, partly because he was slow to clean up the workplace. "Fleming began to tease me about my excessive tidiness," Allison recalled, because "at the end of each day's work I cleaned my bench, put it in order for the next day, and discarded tubes and culture plates for which I had no further use." Fleming, in contrast, hoarded culture plates on his bench until he had no more room to work, and then threw out the samples only after scrutinizing each one to see if it held anything interesting.

One evening in November 1921, as Fleming was tossing out his old specimens, he called Allison over to see a plate with a spot of nasal mucus, cultured two weeks earlier from Flem-

ing's own mucus when the scientist had been suffering from a cold. All over the plate were golden colonies of a harmless airborne bacterium that may have been in dust or blown in through the open window. Remarkably, however, no bacteria had grown on the spot of mucus. More striking, the bacteria around the spot were turning pale and translucent—as though something was seeping out from the mucus and killing them.

Fleming decided to try an experiment: In a flask he made a liquid suspension consisting of saline solution and the golden bacteria—creating a cloudy, yellow, infectious soup. To this he added a small amount of nasal mucus. Within two minutes the flask turned "as clear as water," Allison recalled, signaling that the bacteria had been killed.

The experiment marked the start of a two-year investigation of the bactericidal substance in mucus. To find out whether it was something unique to himself, Fleming collected samples of mucus from other lab workers. These also contained the substance, as did tears, saliva, sputum, pus, blood serum, and the fluid of the lungs and the peritoneum (the membrane lining the abdominal cavity). To replenish

his supplies of experimental material, Fleming sometimes paid boys who cleaned the lab—and even asked "unwary visitors," Allison remembered—to contribute tears, coaxed out with a little lemon juice. In his thoroughness, Fleming had Allison collect nonhuman tears as well, from horses, cows, hens, and 50 species in the London Zoo. The antibacterial substance was present in all of them. As Fleming learned, it was a powerful toxin, capable of destroying 75 percent of the 104 strains of airborne bacteria in his collection.

Although Fleming wrote a paper on his discovery and published it in the 1922 *Proceedings of the Royal Society of London*, its importance was not fully honored for many years. One sign of this neglect is that Fleming himself, nominated to the Royal Society in 1923, was not accepted until 1943. Today, lysozyme is recognized as an important part of a many-layered system of defenses that ward off common bacterial infections.

The ability to kill bacteria—but kill them selectively—is essential. From the moment of birth, humans are bathed in potentially threatening organisms. The body kills off some of them, but it nevertheless tolerates a lush garden of "friendly" bacteria on the surface of the skin, in the throat and nasal passages, in the eyes, and around the genital organs. These

Guardian with an Appetite

The immune system's most versatile performers are the white blood cells called phagocytes. Known in their immature form as monocytes and in their mature form as macrophages, they patrol, scavenge, attack, and destroy invaders, send for help, and remove debris. Their technique for disposing of unwanted material is simple but dramatic: They consume it.

The sequence of photographs at right shows a macrophage engulfing a dead, bloated red blood cell in a scene that occurs billions of times a day in the human body. The actual breaking down of the cell will take place inside the macrophage, where enzymes go to work digesting cellular components. The entire process can take up to several hours.

When the digested matter is a microorganism such as a bacterium, a macrophage will go through a more complex procedure (*pages* 62-63) that helps alert other white cells to the presence of invaders. Also in the macrophage repertory is the ability to secrete different types of chemicals with a range of functions—from attracting more phagocytes and other immune cells to a site of infection, to destroying tumors and stimulating the production of blood cells.

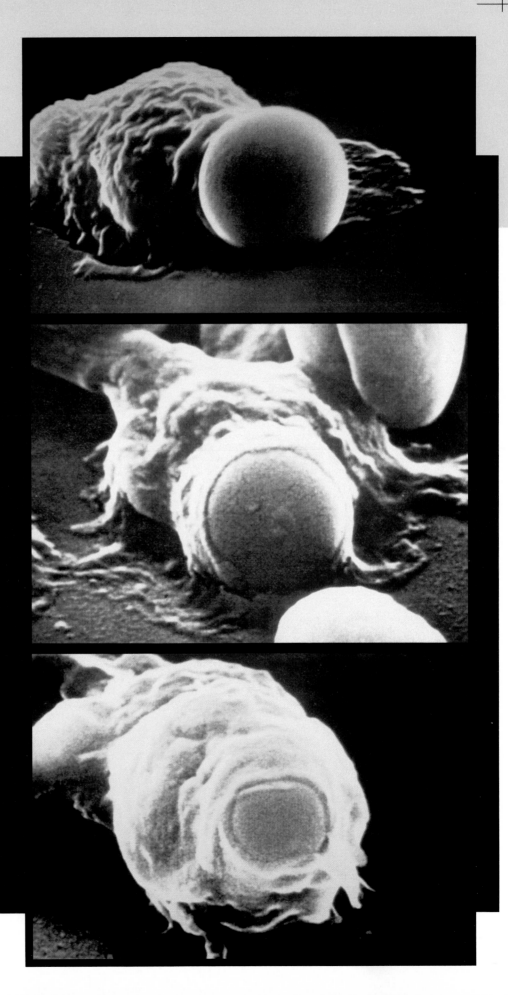

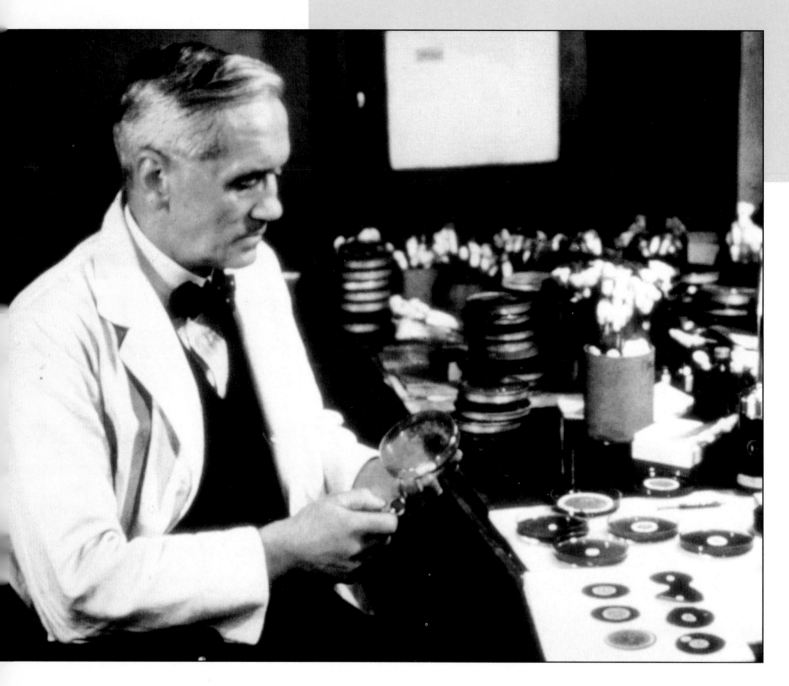

tame bacteria may help to prevent infection by other types, just as a thick grass lawn helps to prevent the growth of weeds. At death, when the body no longer produces lysozyme or other defensive organisms, the balance between friendly and unfriendly organisms ends, and hostile ones rapidly invade and dismantle the body.

Harmful bacteria represent only one type of threat that the body must arm itself against. Indeed, those elements of the defensive system such as macrophages and complement proteins that are effective in attacking bacteria and other relatively sizable foreign matter in the bloodstream are not nearly as skilled at handling invasions of the tiny organic packages known as viruses. Measuring only a few billionths of a meter in diameter—too small to be seen by most microscopes—and consisting of no more than a core of genetic material surrounded by a protein coat, viruses nevertheless constitute one of the

Alexander Fleming *(left)*, known primarily for his work with penicillin, expanded knowledge of the immune system arsenal with his 1921 discovery of lysozyme, a class of antibacterial chemicals present in various bodily fluids. A tireless experimenter, Fleming found that lysozyme is present in a wide range of organic substances, from egg white to turnip juice.

body's most insidious foes, infecting cells and hijacking the cellular machinery to mass-produce themselves. They have been linked to illnesses as benign as the common cold and as malignant as AIDS and are notoriously adept at avoiding defenses. Yet even the virus has enemies. In particular, viruses can be attacked by a general-purpose substance in the blood first identified in the 1950s. Its discoverers were two virologists—a Scot named Alick Isaacs, director of the World Influenza Center in London, and his Swiss colleague, Jean Lindenmann.

Isaacs and Lindenmann learned about the substance through experiments conducted on fresh eggs. They injected a small amount of flu virus (weakened by heating) through the egg membranes into the chicken embryos within. The eggs responded by producing quantities of a protein that Isaacs and Lindenmann successfully purified. It seemed to cling to virus particles and interfere with their replication process, so Isaacs named it interferon. If new eggs were injected with a small amount of this material, the researchers found, they were better able to resist infection: Interferon provided a defensive boost.

Buoyed by these results, Isaacs and

Lindenmann had great hopes of developing an antiviral medicine for humans based on interferon, but despite a decade of effort, they met with no success—in part because interferon was soon found to be species specific, complicating the process of producing supplies of interferon for use against different viral strains. Isaacs died in 1967 at the age of 45, but since then other scientists have made further progress, even to the extent of developing interferon treatments for cancers known to be caused by viral agents.

With the discovery of interferon, the main elements of the immune system—both interior and exterior—had been identified, but still being worked out was one of immunity's most important features: the mechanism by which the body distinguishes friend from foe. Researchers had long been mystified, for example, by the question of how a lymphocyte such as a cytotoxic T cell—also called a killer T cell—prowling the bloodstream and looking for prey could differentiate between one of the body's healthy cells and a seemingly identical traitor harboring a virus within. It has taken more than 30 years for scientists to reach a satisfactory understanding. The first breakthrough came in the early 1950s, with the work of a British researcher, Peter Medawar, and a key

insight from Australian virologist Macfarlane Burnet. The system of cellular identity checks they helped to uncover is remarkable.

Born in Brazil to British parents in 1915, Medawar studied at an elite prep school in England and won top honors in zoology at Magdalen College, Oxford. During World War II he joined a British military research unit treating men with war injuries, particularly victims of fires and pilots whose planes had been shot down. The team was trying to develop a way to remove skin—the most essential defense against infection—from healthy donors and graft it to burn victims who had lost their own. But the group found that the skin grafts were always rejected or sloughed off within two weeks. After analyzing the patterns of rejection, Medawar and a colleague, Thomas Gibson of the Glasgow Royal Infirmary, concluded that the source of trouble was not a local bacterial reaction at the point of surgery, but something systemic. Some elemental process of the immune system was identifying the transplants as foreign and attacking them. Medawar went on to investigate how and why the immune system might be producing this effect.

Following the work of other scientists in the field, Medawar began conducting experiments with rabbits and mice at Oxford. He concluded that many independent factors were involved in tissue rejection, but he was not able to come up with a clear picture. Meanwhile, at the University of Wisconsin, American researcher Ray Owen had discovered that nonidentical cattle twins—that is, ones that had shared the same uterus but did not have the same genetic makeup—had mixtures of each other's blood cells but did not develop antibodies against the foreign cells of the twin. Burnet picked up on the study, realizing that it held significance for the question of immunological tolerance. He brought up the subject in a book published in 1949, noting that, based on Owen's findings, the immune system must be partly inherited and partly acquired in the embryo after conception. It was, therefore, capable of modification. Upon reading Burnet's hypothesis, Medawar was inspired to put it to the test.

Along with his assistant, Rupert Billingham, and zoology student Leslie Brent, Medawar undertook some new studies on several strains of mice. In a series of meticulous experiments completed in 1953, the researchers demonstrated that it was possible to fool one mouse's immune system into accepting cells from another as self.

Specifically, Medawar showed that white mice could be made to tolerate skin grafts from brown mice if cells from the brown mice had been injected into the embryonic sacs of the white mice. This caused the immune systems of the white mice, in effect, to learn to see two distinct identities as self. Later it became clear that this tolerance could be induced even as late as the first day after birth. Finally, Medawar repeated the experiment in chick embryos, proving that the pattern is common to animals other than mice. In 1960 he won the Nobel Prize, which he shared with Macfarlane Burnet.

During the 1960s, scientists building on this work identified a group of genes that control the graft-rejection process. The genes they found came to be known as the major histocompatibility complex (MHC), after their role in skin grafts (histo refers to tissue). But while this discovery arose from skin research, it soon became clear that the proteins arising from the MHC genes affect all aspects of the immune system.

Researchers discovered that MHC controls immunity based in the blood, as well as skin-tissue compatibility. Investigating patterns within

families, they also found that every individual inherits two distinct genetic instruction sets for creating an MHC system, one from the mother and one from the father. The researchers involved in these studies worked out a relatively simple classification scheme in which the father's genetic contributions were labeled a and b (one from his father and one from his mother), and the mother's c and d (one from each of her parents). It was assumed that each child would therefore inherit one of four basic histocompatibility types: ac, ad, bc, or bd. Children with identical types—say, a brother and sister with ac type—would thus be more likely to accept tissue transplants from one another than children with nonidentical types. This hypothesis raised a hope in the mid-1960s that it might be possible to organize blood and tissue immune responses into readily identifiable categories, but, unfortunately, that was not to be. There was much more variability than had originally been assumed, and many exceptions to what had been an appealingly simple set of rules.

The full complexity of the MHC system became clear as immunologists focused on killer T cells, the enforcers that attack sick or infected cells in the bloodstream. The MHC system plays an important dual role in stimulating T cells: It both incites and limits their destructive action. For

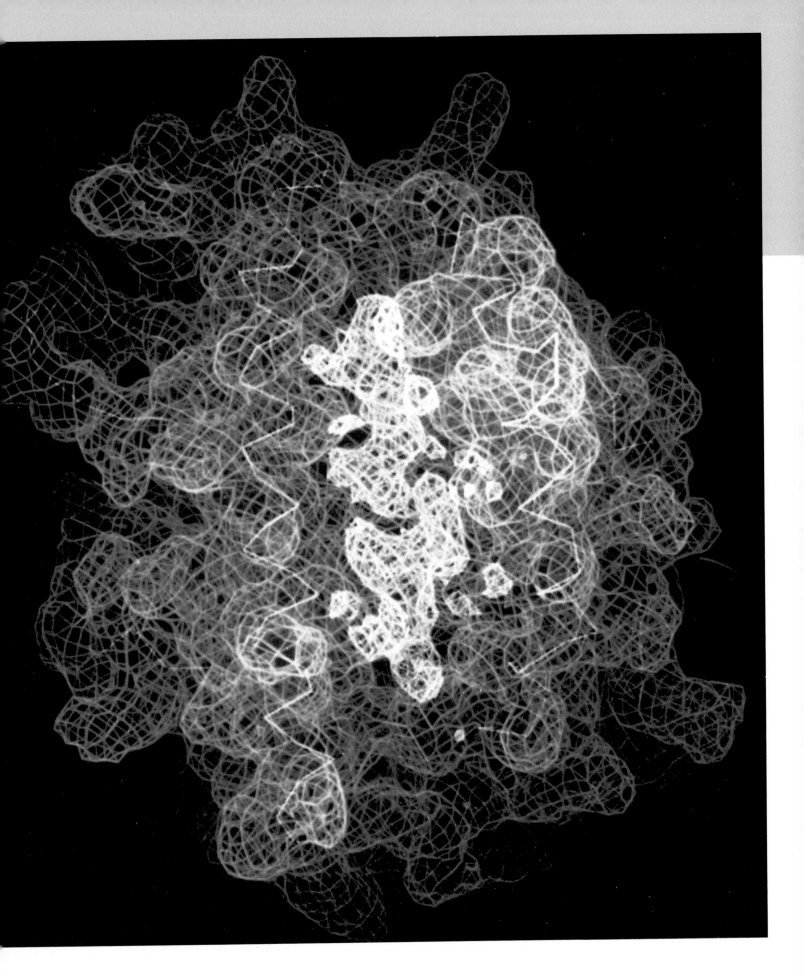

example, a T cell will attack a virus-infected cell viciously—but only if the T cell detects the presence of an antigen, or nonself material, and at the same time detects an MHC protein containing the flag that signals "self" attached to the target. In other words, before it attacks, the T cell must "see" two elements on each target. The practical effect is that the T cells will not attack just anything that appears unusual, but only things that have been specifically tagged by the body's MHC proteins as alien. This control helps to prevent the body from releasing too many T cells, which might deplete friendly elements of the body.

For more than a decade, experts debated whether the T cell sees the MHC self flag and the nonself antigen as a single unit or as two separate entities. The debate ended abruptly in 1987 when a group of researchers at Harvard crystallized an MHC protein and captured its image with x-rays. The structure was so clear, according to Harvard researcher Jack Strominger, that there could be no confusion: The MHC presents one point for T cells to scan for identity. What the x-ray image showed was that the MHC molecule is a structure with a single cleft, or groove, on the surface, to which an antigen fragment will be bound when the target cell is infected. This whole structure is what

is recognized as foreign by T cells.

With their microscopic army, humans have defended themselves throughout the ages against attack by viruses, bacteria, and even larger, more complex microorganisms such as parasites. The safeguards are remarkably thorough. But there is one type of invasion that causes the body to lay down its armor, one that has defeated even the strongest bastions of the immune system. In fact, the fate of the human species rests on the ability of this invader to overpower all defenses: It is the sperm.

From the female immune system's perspective, the male sperm looks a lot like an invader. Roughly 200 to 500 million of these microscopic or-

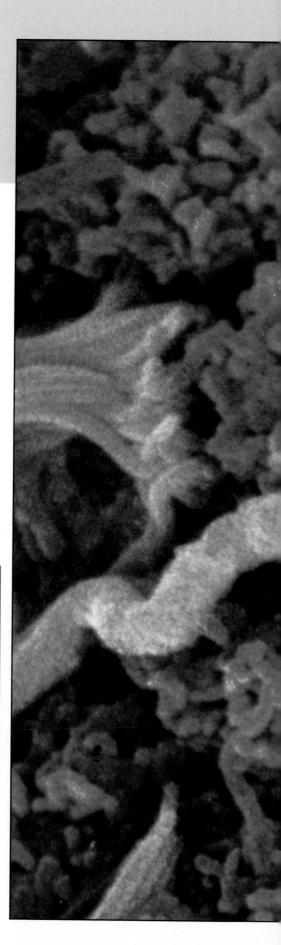

A single human sperm cell on its way through the reproductive tract encounters defensive measures designed to thwart foreign material. Hairlike cilia create adverse currents that repel most antigens but that sperm can swim against. Although secretions of the mucous membrane *(red)* also stave off invaders, during ovulation the mucus thins enough to allow some sperm to get through. A coating *(orange)* at the head of the sperm contains enzymes that will help break down a protective barrier of nutrient material surrounding the sperm's ultimate goal—the egg.

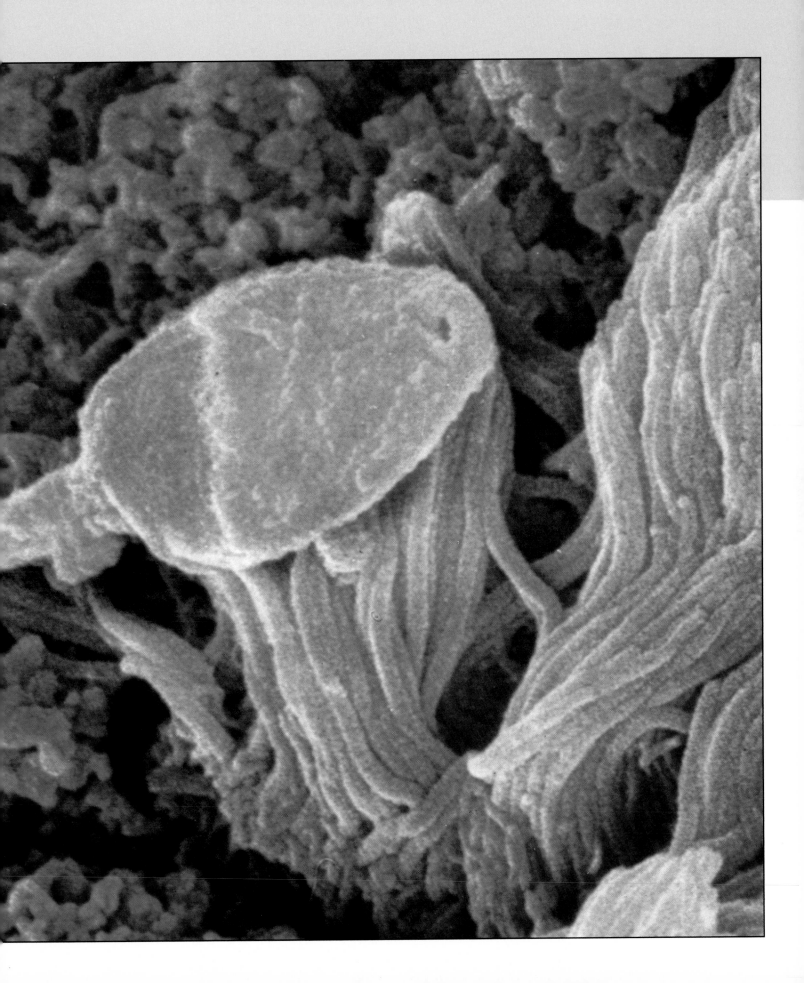

ganisms enter a woman's body during sexual intercourse and swim toward the uterus and fallopian tubes. They all strive to fuse with an egg and produce an embryo, but only one can succeed. On its surface, each sperm carries the male's proteins, identifying it to the woman's system as nonself, a target for attack. Perhaps 100 million are killed immediately by acids and white cells in the protective mucus of the vagina. It is essential to species survival, however, that some sperm get through. To this end, mammals have developed an elaborate pattern of mechanisms to permit roughly 1,000 sperm to enter the uterus, and a few hundred the fallopian tubes, so that one can unite with the egg.

Ordinarily, an invasion of the magnitude of a sperm infusion would produce inflammation in the uterus, but the seminal fluid that carries the sperm holds a soothing substance that prevents this response and also helps shield the sperm from attack.

After fertilization, however, inflammation does occur, with beneficial effects. As the irritated fallopian tubes swell, they narrow, holding the fertilized egg in place as it descends to the uterus and thereby guarding against miscarriage.

As the embryo grows, it develops an immune identity only half derived from the mother, so that by all rights it too should trigger attacks by the mother's immune system. However, the placenta—which forms where the mucous membrane of the uterus meets the membranes of the fetus— serves as a semipermeable barrier, helping to screen out the mother's T cells but at the same time allowing beneficial antibodies from the mother, as well as nutrients, to reach the fetus. Researchers have yet to understand precisely how all this is accom-

plished, but clearly the mother's self-protective forces are held in check sufficiently to allow this new, foreign organism to thrive.

Miraculously, then, what started as an embryonic cluster of cells with no immunity of its own becomes, by birth, a person who has begun to raise up an army of internal defenders. In time, this immune system must learn to identify and distinguish the brand new ''self'' it protects from all other organisms, and it must educate itself in great detail about many hostile parasites, bacteria, and viruses in the world outside. Along the way, of course, there are almost always bound to be occasions when the inborn defenses prove insufficient, and outside help becomes necessary. For their part, the efforts throughout history to develop effective forms of such assistance have provided some of the most significant insights into how the body goes about marshaling its defending army.

EQUIPPED FOR THE STRUGGLE

The front-line troops of the immune system are the leukocytes—white blood cells that circulate through the body and garrison a few strategic organs to defend against infectious agents. The cells are generated and transported by the lymphatic system, a network whose primary organs are the bone marrow, where all blood cells arise, and the thymus, where T cells learn to recognize and destroy specific antigens. To ensure that antigens are quickly detected and fought, white blood cells continuously patrol the body, circulating both in the blood and in the clear lymph that moves through the specialized channels called lymphatic vessels.

Some immune cells gather in secondary lymphoid organs, where they work together to recognize and respond to antigens. Foremost are the lymph nodes, filters located at junctions of the lymphatic vessels, and the spleen, which screens foreign matter from the blood. Other clusters of lymphoid tissue include the tonsils and adenoids in the back of the throat; the appendix, located off the large intestine; and Peyer's patches—named for the 17th-century Swiss physician who discovered them—on the wall of the small intestine.

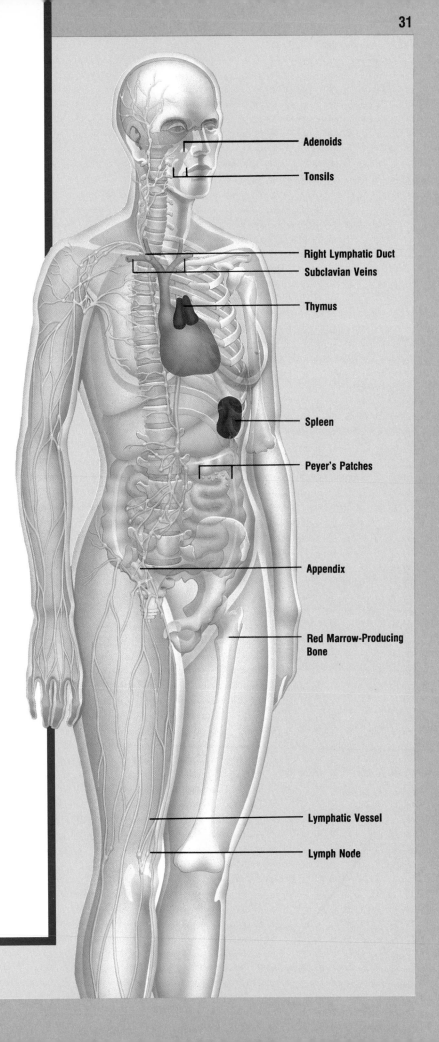

- Adenoids
- Tonsils
- Right Lymphatic Duct
- Subclavian Veins
- Thymus
- Spleen
- Peyer's Patches
- Appendix
- Red Marrow-Producing Bone
- Lymphatic Vessel
- Lymph Node

CREATION IN THE MARROW

Although all bones have a marrow core, only some of them contain red marrow, the source of white blood cells as well as of other blood cells that circulate through the body. Red marrow, a gelatinous jumble of cells, may be found only in the ends of the long bones, such as the thighbone and the upper arm bone, and in the vertebrae, ribs, breastbone, col-larbone, shoulder blades, hipbones, and skull (*far right*).

The progenitors of the circulating cells are known as stem cells. Regulated by a little-understood hormonal mechanism, stem cells differentiate into a variety of specialized immune cells, each with a role to play in the immune response. Some stem cell offspring are large white blood cells, including granulocytes and monocytes, whose purpose is to attack harmful cells and foreign particles. Others are lymphocytes, a class of smaller white blood cells involved in the specific immune response and composed mainly of precursor T cells and B cells (which also have a precursor stage, not shown here).

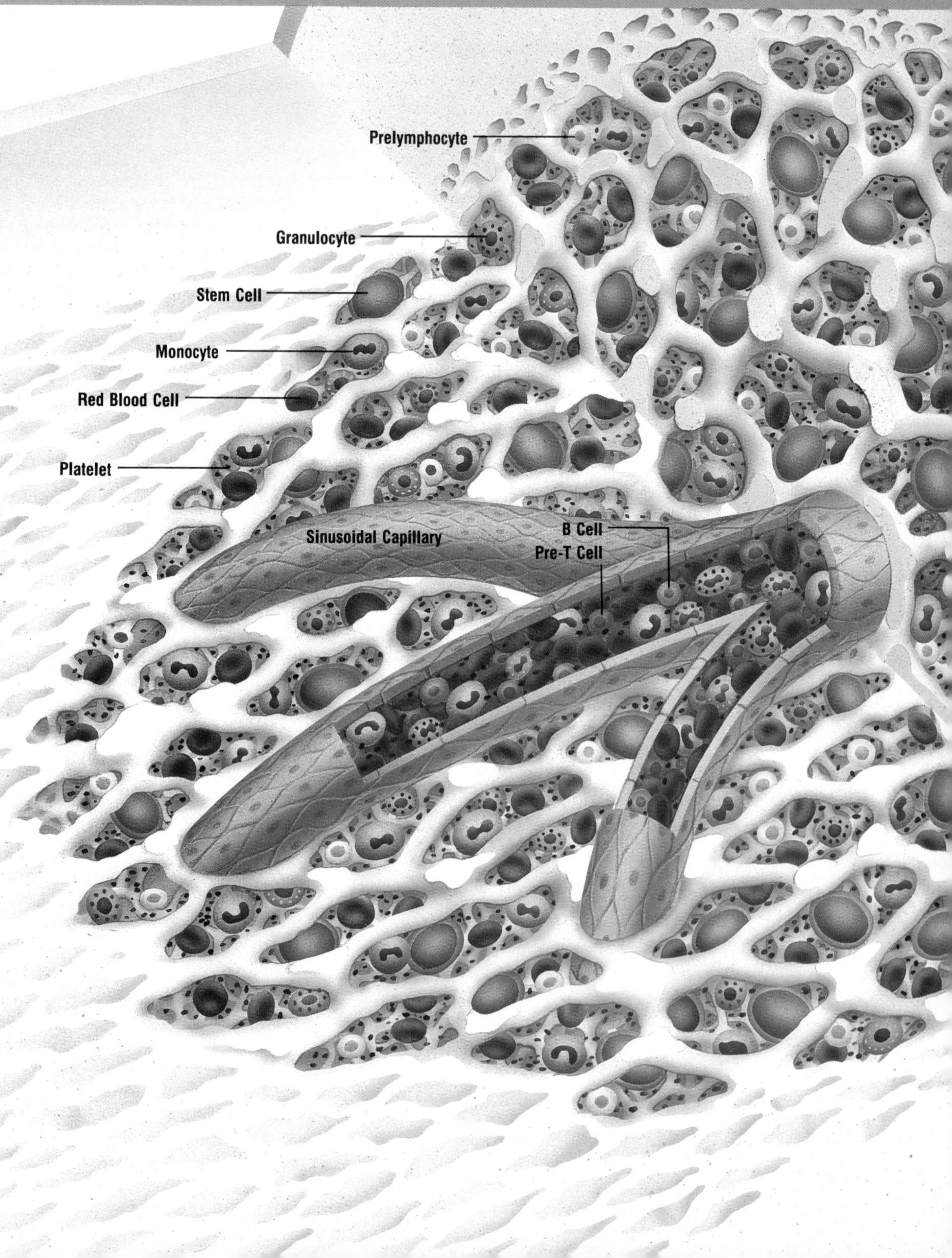

AT THE SOURCE. Inside the hard outer layers of the long bones lies red marrow *(right)*, the well-spring of the circulatory system. Here stem cells divide to produce precursor lymphocytes, which transform themselves into B cells and pre-T cells. Stem cells also differentiate into granulocytes, monocytes, red blood cells, and platelets. The pressure created by the formation of all these new cells pushes them against the wall of the sinusoidal capillary, forcing gaps between the capillary cells; as immune cells pass through into the blood-stream, the capillary walls close behind them.

Prelymphocyte

Granulocyte

Stem Cell

Monocyte

Red Blood Cell

Platelet

Sinusoidal Capillary

B Cell
Pre-T Cell

More than a billion immune cells pour out of the red marrow each day, to replace those that die of old age or are destroyed by other processes.

Granulocytes mature and are ready to fight as soon as they enter the circulatory system. Monocytes, on the other hand, develop into full-fledged macrophages only after they leave the bloodstream to enter tissue. Some lymphocytes must go elsewhere in the lymphatic system to mature and become part of the immune arsenal: Pre-T cells travel to the thymus for a rigorous "education" (*pages* 34-35), and B cells go to the lymph nodes and spleen to await activation by antigens (*pages* 36-37).

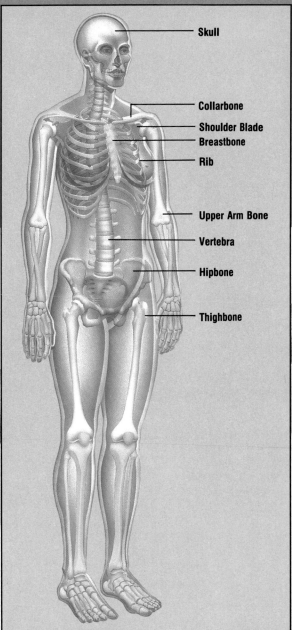

- Skull
- Collarbone
- Shoulder Blade
- Breastbone
- Rib
- Upper Arm Bone
- Vertebra
- Hipbone
- Thighbone

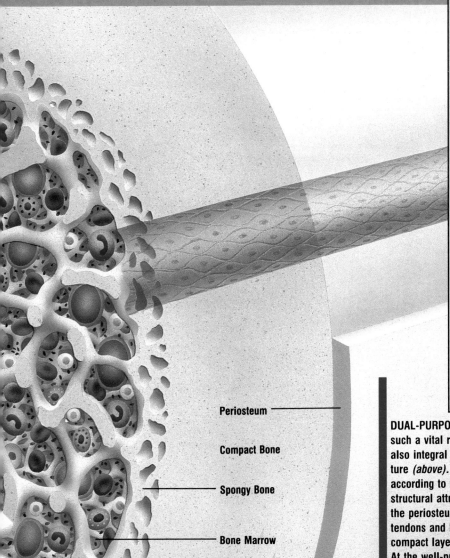

- Periosteum
- Compact Bone
- Spongy Bone
- Bone Marrow

DUAL-PURPOSE BONES. The bones that play such a vital role in the circulatory system are also integral parts of the body's skeletal structure *(above)*. Although they differ in shape according to their function, all share basic structural attributes. The outside of each bone, the periosteum *(left),* forms an anchorage for tendons and ligaments. Next comes a dense, compact layer that gives the bone its strength. At the well-protected, spongy core of the bone lies the blood cell-producing marrow.

TOUGH TRAINING FOR ASPIRING T CELLS

Because of its location high on the heart and beneath the breastbone, the thymus was regarded by the ancient Greeks as the seat of courage and affection. The real function of the two-lobed thymus is more basic: Within its many small lobules, T cells (which get their name from the thymus) are rigorously selected for their functions in the specific immune response. Much of the gland's work is done during childhood, and it begins to atrophy rapidly during late adolescence.

After leaving the bone marrow, a pre-T cell circulates in the blood before migrating to the thymus. There, hormonal activity

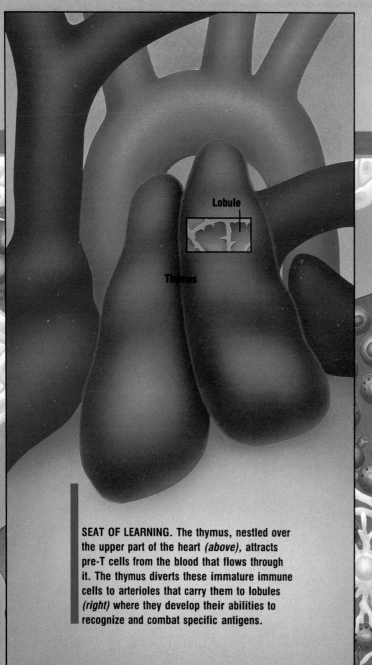

Lobule

Thymus

SEAT OF LEARNING. The thymus, nestled over the upper part of the heart *(above)*, attracts pre-T cells from the blood that flows through it. The thymus diverts these immature immune cells to arterioles that carry them to lobules *(right)* where they develop their abilities to recognize and combat specific antigens.

and cellular interaction cause it to multiply and descend through the cortex and medulla, where it attains the mature form that will identify antigens and infected tissue cells.

A T cell's education involves the development of receptor sites—surface proteins that allow the lymphocytes to react to both antigens and the special MHC molecules that identify the body's own tissue cells. Myriad varieties of receptors appear in the first stages of T cell maturation, but only a few receptor types make it through the ruthless selection process (*below*), which builds vital safeguards into the immune system. T cells that recognize only antigens and not self-MHC molecules would be ineffectual, unable to deal with infected body cells. But too strong a reaction to self-MHC is not suitable either; a T cell that treats normal body-cell proteins the same way it treats antigens would attack healthy tissues, creating autoimmune diseases. Only cells that demonstrate a partial affinity for self-MHC, thus being able to recognize a combination of self-MHC and an antigen, make the grade. A scant one percent of pre-T cells entering the thymus survive the test and emerge as mature, antigen-specific T cells; the rest are destroyed there.

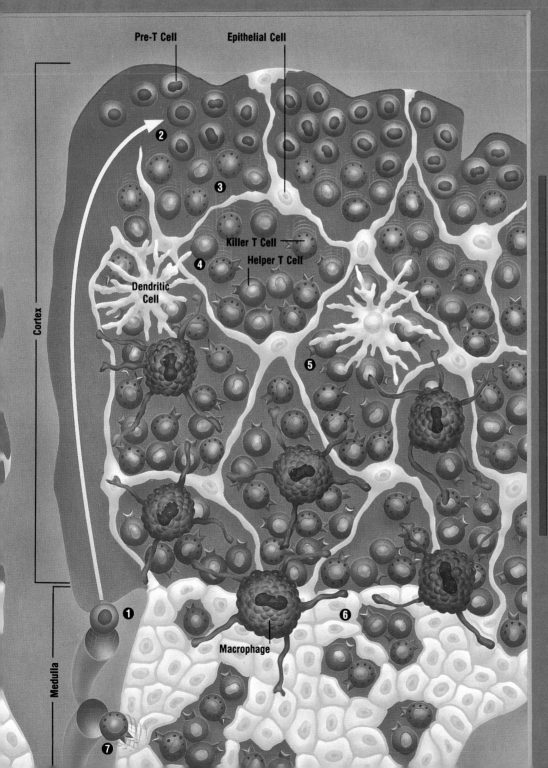

Pre-T Cell
Epithelial Cell
Killer T Cell
Helper T Cell
Dendritic Cell
Cortex
Medulla
Macrophage

RITE OF PASSAGE. The arteriole delivers pre-T cells about halfway up each lobule *(1)*, and they migrate to the top of the cortex *(2)*. As they begin to descend through a web of epithelial cells, they divide repeatedly *(3)*, giving rise to families of helper T cells and cytotoxic, or killer, T cells. Specific genes within these cells randomly switch on, causing the expression of antigen receptors on the cells' surfaces *(4)*.

The newly equipped T cells then test themselves against dendritic cells, macrophages, and epithelial cells that carry self-MHC *(5)*. Too poor or too close a fit triggers self-destruction and removal by macrophages; T cells that partially recognize the self-MHC and antigen pass the test *(6)*. These surviving T cells travel into the medulla, then exit by way of a venule *(7)*, passing back into the bloodstream ready to battle antigens.

KEY ROLES FOR THE LYMPH NODES AND SPLEEN

B cells generated in the bone marrow reach their full antigen-fighting potential in the lymph nodes and spleen, secondary organs of the lymphatic system that filter antigens from the blood and lymph. The appearance of antigens in these organs triggers the transformation of B cells into plasma cells, which will in turn produce customized antibodies that travel to infection areas.

As the bloodstream circulates immune cells through arteries and capillaries to body tissue, the yellowish liquid part of the blood, called plasma (which is different from plasma cells), seeps out of the capillaries of the circulatory system to transport oxygen, nutrients, and immune cells into the interstices,

LYMPHATIC FLUID. The web of tiny blood capillaries that carries oxygen and nutrients *(below, top left)* also releases a clear, yellowish fluid into the spaces between tissue cells. This fluid, carrying immune cells as well as antigenic particles, enters the lymphatic system by seeping through the single-cell walls of lymph capillaries. The capillaries converge to form larger lymphatic vessels (equipped with one-way valves to prevent backflow), which carry their contents—now called lymph—to lymph nodes for filtration.

FILTERING CENTERS. Lymph nodes, lying along the lymphatic vessels, contain several lobules and a network of internal channels *(below).* In each lobule the lymph percolates through a cortex with an outer layer of B cells and an inner layer of T cells. Antigens in the lymph interact with B cells and T cells, initiating an immune response. T cells specific to the antigen, along with other immune cells, leave through an outgoing lymphatic vessel to battle the infection in tissue cells.

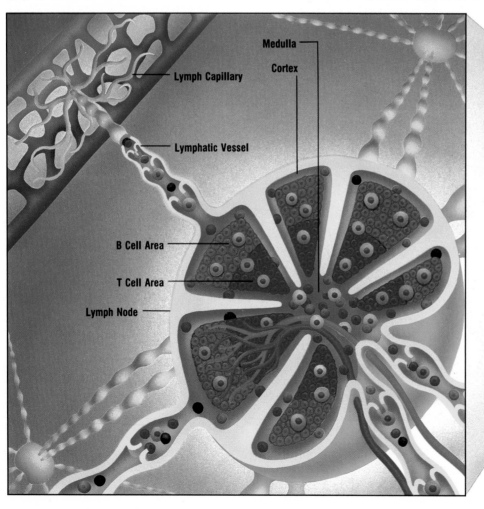

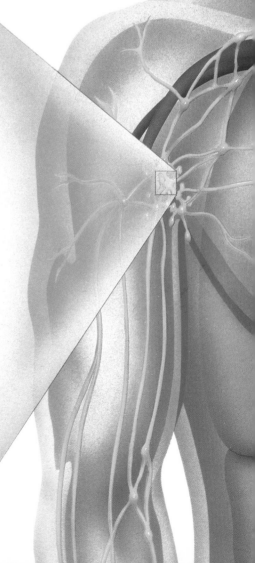

Lymph Capillary

Medulla

Cortex

Lymphatic Vessel

B Cell Area

T Cell Area

Lymph Node

or spaces, between the tissue cells. This interstitial fluid surrounds the cells with everything that they need to live; in addition, it provides a medium for communication, by the exchange of chemicals between cells. The interstitial fluid is also important to the immune system, because white blood cells roaming in the fluid can encounter and begin to fight antigens there (*pages* 62-63).

A specialized network of lymphatic vessels continually drains the interstitial fluid for filtration and further use. Tiny lymphatic capillaries, with walls only a single cell thick, allow antigen-bearing fluid to enter from the interstitial space. The lymphatic system collects this lymph, filters it through lymph nodes, and then returns it to the blood. Unlike the blood system, which is driven by the pumping of the heart, the lymphatic system is powered by muscle contractions throughout the body, both voluntary and involuntary. These contractions enable it to move about three quarts of lymph each day from the interstitial space back into the bloodstream.

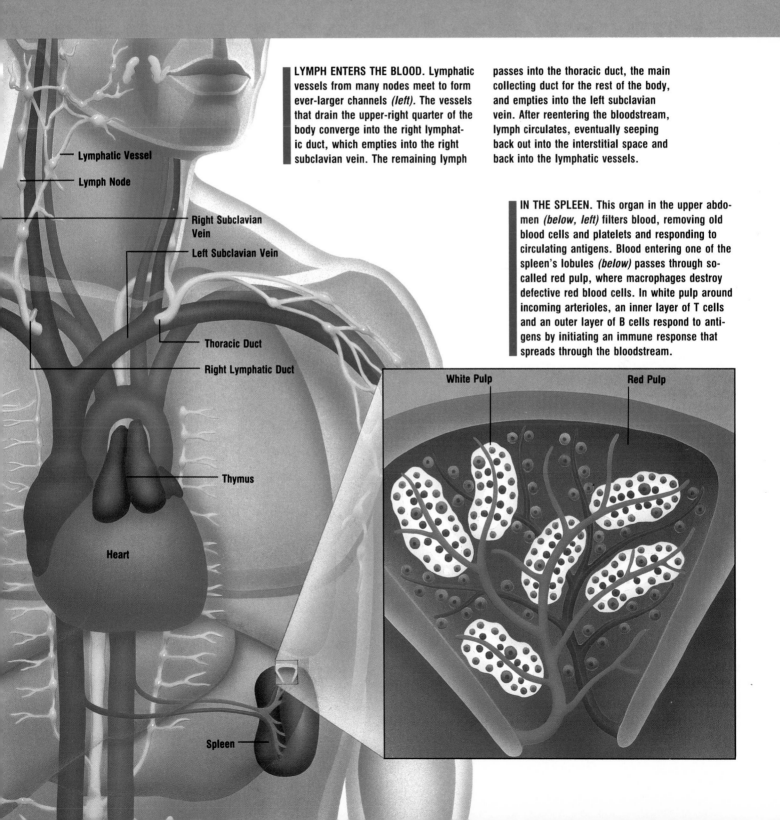

LYMPH ENTERS THE BLOOD. Lymphatic vessels from many nodes meet to form ever-larger channels *(left).* The vessels that drain the upper-right quarter of the body converge into the right lymphatic duct, which empties into the right subclavian vein. The remaining lymph passes into the thoracic duct, the main collecting duct for the rest of the body, and empties into the left subclavian vein. After reentering the bloodstream, lymph circulates, eventually seeping back out into the interstitial space and back into the lymphatic vessels.

IN THE SPLEEN. This organ in the upper abdomen *(below, left)* filters blood, removing old blood cells and platelets and responding to circulating antigens. Blood entering one of the spleen's lobules *(below)* passes through so-called red pulp, where macrophages destroy defective red blood cells. In white pulp around incoming arterioles, an inner layer of T cells and an outer layer of B cells respond to antigens by initiating an immune response that spreads through the bloodstream.

Lymphatic Vessel

Lymph Node

Right Subclavian Vein

Left Subclavian Vein

Thoracic Duct

Right Lymphatic Duct

Thymus

Heart

Spleen

White Pulp

Red Pulp

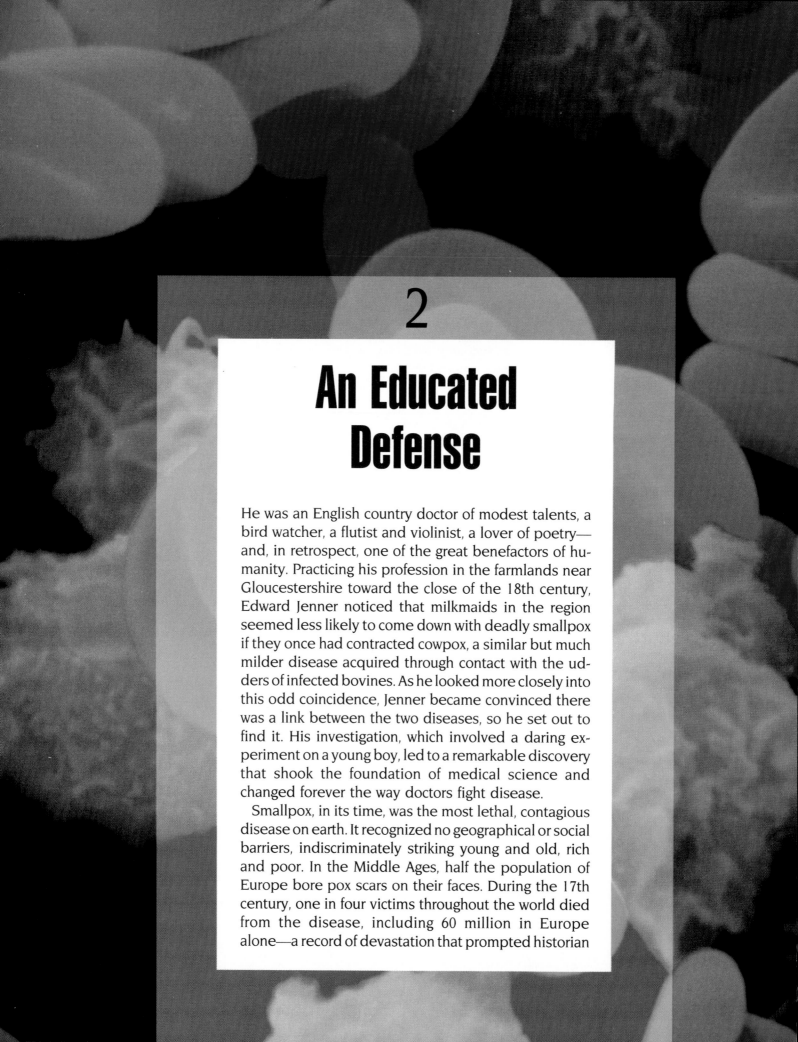

2

An Educated Defense

He was an English country doctor of modest talents, a bird watcher, a flutist and violinist, a lover of poetry—and, in retrospect, one of the great benefactors of humanity. Practicing his profession in the farmlands near Gloucestershire toward the close of the 18th century, Edward Jenner noticed that milkmaids in the region seemed less likely to come down with deadly smallpox if they once had contracted cowpox, a similar but much milder disease acquired through contact with the udders of infected bovines. As he looked more closely into this odd coincidence, Jenner became convinced there was a link between the two diseases, so he set out to find it. His investigation, which involved a daring experiment on a young boy, led to a remarkable discovery that shook the foundation of medical science and changed forever the way doctors fight disease.

Smallpox, in its time, was the most lethal, contagious disease on earth. It recognized no geographical or social barriers, indiscriminately striking young and old, rich and poor. In the Middle Ages, half the population of Europe bore pox scars on their faces. During the 17th century, one in four victims throughout the world died from the disease, including 60 million in Europe alone—a record of devastation that prompted historian

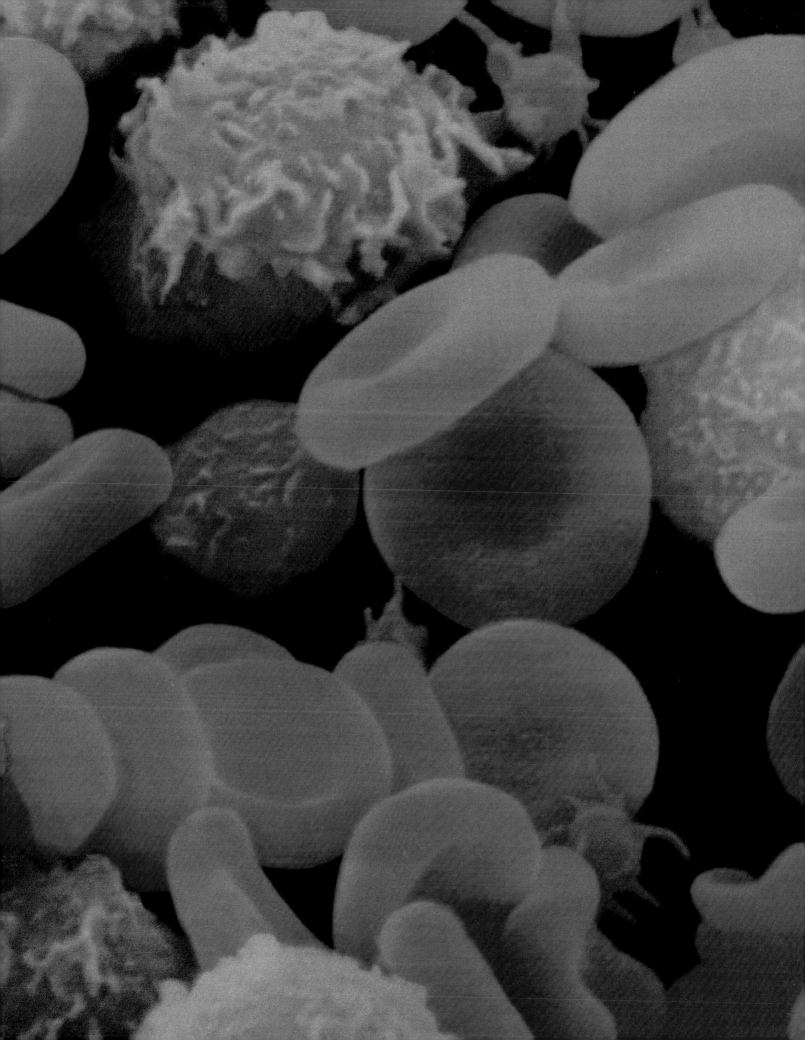

Thomas Macaulay 200 years later to dub smallpox "the most terrible of all the ministers of death."

The pernicious germ worked its evil from the inside out. Starting in the respiratory system, the virus took up residence in its victim's lymph glands and liver, then multiplied inside cells until it burst forth to invade the skin. After a few days, lesions appeared on the mucous membranes of the mouth and throat. Fever and muscle aches racked the body, which after eight to 10 days was covered with a rash that, in extreme cases, caused large amounts of skin to peel away. The rash developed into painful blisters, and these in turn gave way to oozing, pus-filled ulcers from which the infectious virus jumped to clothes, bed linens, and even dust particles, there to lie in wait for a new host.

For healthy people hoping to avoid this agonizing pestilence, physicians of Jenner's day used a procedure, called ingrafting or "buying the pox," introduced in England from Turkey earlier in the century. Doctors would scratch the skin of the person's arm several times with the tip of a needle or knife, then place the dried scab or pus from the sore of a smallpox victim over the fresh cuts. A few days later, the patient would come down with a case of smallpox but would usually suffer only minor body sores and no more than a few days of fever

before the disease relented, never to return again. (The principle of ingrafting may actually have originated in China, where instead of using scabs, physicians blew infected matter into the nose through a silver tube, using the left nostril for males and the right for females.)

Jenner, however, had severe misgivings about buying the pox, even though the method often proved successful. Years before, as one of several children in his village who had escaped the disease, he had undergone the excruciating procedure himself at the hands of an ignorant doctor. Young Jenner was bled repeatedly and starved to "purge" his system, then treated with the scab of a smallpox victim and forced to remain in a stable. Within a week he developed a bright red rash and a fever, both of which disappeared after three days. As smallpox went, the case was a mild one. But it took the weakened boy nearly a month to recover from the combined effects of the illness and the diabolical treatment.

As he tended to his patients in Gloucestershire, Jenner resolved to find a safer, less painful approach to warding off the disease. Perhaps, he thought, something transmitted from

cows infected with cowpox to human hands shielded the milkmaids from the human version of the sickness. Jenner began roaming from farm to farm in search of cowpox outbreaks, looking for clues. Farmers thought he was crazy and chased Jenner from their land, yet for 18 years he stubbornly carried on.

Finally, in May 1796, Jenner decided to try an extraordinary experiment. He took pus from a cowpox sore on the hand of a milkmaid named Sarah Nelmes and scratched it into the arm of a healthy eight-year-old boy, James Phipps. The boy spent one uncomfortable night, but he was perfectly fine the following day. Two months later, in a highly risky move, Jenner again subjected the youngster to infection, this time from a smallpox sore. Just as the doctor had hoped, the patient showed no sign of illness. Indeed, young Phipps lived to be an old man, deliberately exposing himself to smallpox another 20 times over the course of his life, to prove his immunity.

As it turned out, Jenner was not the first to use the procedure; two decades before his experiment, a cattle dealer in the area named Benjamin Jesty had successfully inoculated his wife and three sons with cowpox to ward off smallpox. Jenner, however, was the first to recognize the importance of the discovery, to study it

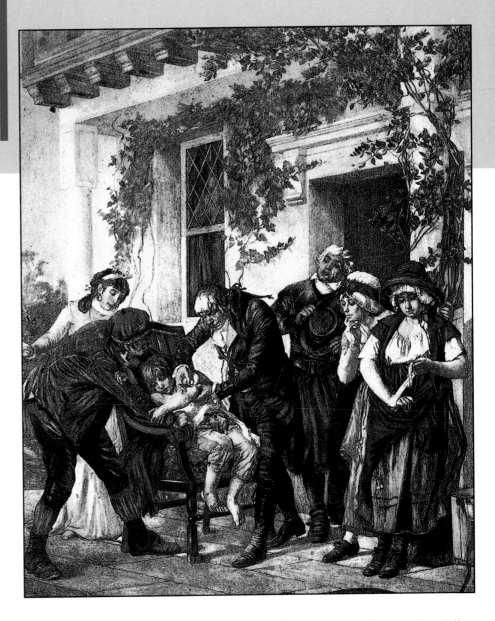

In 18th-century England, Edward Jenner scratches pus from a cowpox sore into the arm of healthy James Phipps. As a result, the boy developed lifelong immunity to smallpox, a similar but much deadlier disease. Jenner's procedure, which he dubbed vaccination, demonstrated the body's ability to "remember" certain diseases and fend off future incursions.

through systematic experimentation, and to spread its use to the general population. He called his technique vaccination, taking the name from the Latin *vacca* for "cow."

Like many of history's great achievements, the breakthrough was greeted not by enthusiastic cheers but largely by indifference and criticism. Religious purists condemned the practice of vaccination, in one case labeling it "a daring and profane violation of our holy order." His colleagues blasted Jenner for using unscientific, life-threatening techniques—breaches serious enough to warrant expulsion from their medical society. The discovery prompted some opponents to organize a society of antivaccinationists. Over time, however, Jenner became recognized for having helped rid the earth of one of humankind's most terrible scourges. Today, vaccines against a host of diseases—including polio, measles, mumps, typhus and typhoid fever, cholera, rubella, yellow fever, and rabies—all have been developed on principles he brought to light.

What Jenner had unknowingly tapped was the mystery of acquired immunity, the body's remarkable ability to develop specific protection

against foreign microorganisms, protection that remains on call to repel future attacks. Only in recent years have scientists begun to piece together the full capability of this precision fighting force. Throughout the body, billions of cells of various classes are linked in a complex communications network, able to pass information back and forth through secretions of special chemicals. These cells can create profiles of invading organisms by "reading" patterns of molecules

on their outer membranes, then kill the intruders and file away blueprints for later reference—attacking the invaders more efficiently with each successive assault.

Although he never knew it, Jenner was using a live virus (cowpox) whose outer membrane happened to be so similar to the smallpox virus that the

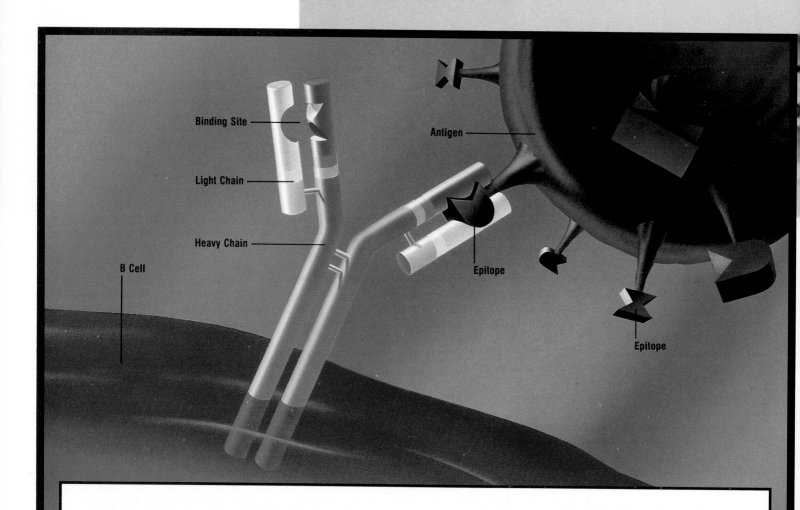

Binding Site

Light Chain

Heavy Chain

B Cell

Antigen

Epitope

Epitope

A Lock for Every Key

One of the immune system's most resourceful defenders, B cells owe their keen powers for recognizing a wide variety of enemies to Y-shaped proteins called receptors dotting their outer membrane. When a receptor encounters a foreign substance, it examines the shape of epitopes—molecular appendages—protruding from the invader's surface. If an epitope's "key" matches the receptor's "lock," the two will form a bond.

The receptor's secret lies in its structure. Each of its arms, shown above as identical tubular segments, is actually a chain of amino acids. The long, angled sections anchoring the receptor are known as heavy chains; the shorter pieces near the top are called light chains. Together, they form a binding site, whose shape is determined by the sequence of amino acids within distinct regions represented here by colored bands. The shifting of a few amino acids in these regions can create a receptor suitable for an entirely different antigen.

Unlike an ordinary gene, which is made up of fixed segments of genetic material, the genes that code for the amino acid chains of a B cell receptor are more random. A receptor's light chain contains several thousand possible amino acid sequences, its heavy chain more than two million. Combined, the two chains can yield billions of possible types of receptors—each capable of matching a different epitope.

Taking aim at a single antigen is the first step toward destroying an entire army of them. Once a receptor has locked onto an epitope, it triggers a chain reaction of sorts in the B cell that culminates in the mass production of antibodies. Virtually identical to the B cell receptor itself, the antibodies will travel through the blood vessels and the lymphatic system, locking onto any antigens that match the first.

body's immune system could not tell the two apart. Today scientists know that such incursions into the body activate millions of specialized white blood cells. Some of these cells, called lymphocytes, release the tiny free-floating proteins known as antibodies, which patrol the body's fluids like eager scouts. Antibodies either neutralize intruders directly or, after marking them for easy identification, hold them at bay until other warrior cells of the immune system arrive to destroy them.

Because the cowpox virus, though outwardly similar to smallpox, is not well adapted to human hosts, it is easily vanquished and rendered harmless by the body's defenses. Once put on alert to an intruder, however, the immune system never forgets. After a cowpox invasion, some of the custom-made lymphocytes produced during the mobilization remain in the body for long periods, sometimes for life. If deadly smallpox ever comes calling, these cells quickly rally to generate more antibodies—as many as 30,000 per second—each one designed specifically to attack poxlike viruses. Not even the potent smallpox virus can withstand the destructive power of the lymphocytes once

they have been primed by the lesser cowpox microbe.

Jenner's discovery was of monumental medical importance, but he was hardly the first to ponder the body's amazing ability to build up resistance to disease. Long before English villagers began buying the pox, one of the Vedic Sanskrit books dating from 1200 BC described how to perform an inoculation, probably for smallpox: "[P]ut fluid from the pustules onto the point of a needle, and introduce it into the arm, mixing the fluid with the blood. A fever will be produced, but this illness will be very mild and need inspire no alarm."

The ancient Greeks also recognized that people who had recovered from some diseases would not get them again. In his description of the mysterious plague that killed almost a quarter of the population of Athens in 430 BC, the historian Thucydides wrote that the sick and dying found "most compassion" in those who had recovered, "for the same man was never attacked twice—never at least fatally." And in AD 541, the historian Procopius wrote of a bubonic plague pandemic that had swept the Byzantine Empire: "It left neither island nor cave nor mountain ridge which had human inhabitants, and if it had passed by any land, either not affecting the men there or touching them in indifferent fashion, still at a later

time it came back; then those who dwelt roundabout this land, whom formerly it had afflicted most sorely, it did not touch at all."

For the most part, however, from biblical times through the Middle Ages, infectious disease was associated with vengeful gods, punishment for sin, and black magic. Even after Jenner published his findings in 1798, progress in developing new ways to fight disease was slow. Doctors realized that a healthy patient could gain protection against a disease from some agent transferred from an infected person, yet no one knew what that mysterious substance might be. Gradually, answers began to emerge during the 1870s from the burgeoning field of bacteriology, most notably from the respective laboratories of two men now regarded as titans of science: German pathologist Robert Koch and French chemist Louis Pasteur. With painstaking research that was often one part genius and two parts hit-or-miss, these scientists vastly extended the principles Jenner had brought to light almost a century earlier. Although Koch and Pasteur despised each other, trading insults in a feud that was part of the larger Franco-Prussian animosity at the time, their

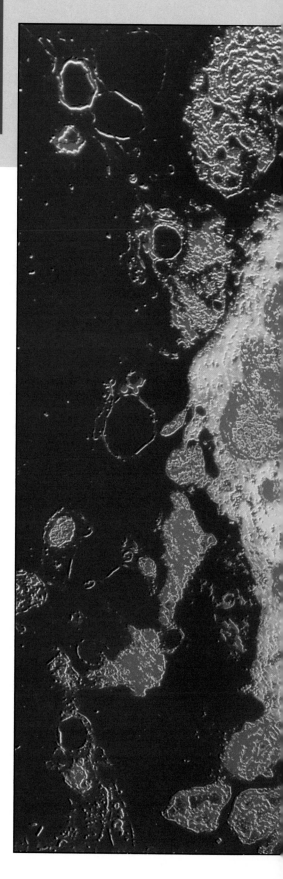

A false-color electron micrograph reveals the internal structure of a plasma cell, the mature form of B cell that handles antibody production. Antibodies are synthesized outside the nucleus, in the surrounding cytoplasm *(yellow)*. A single plasma cell can release as many as 30,000 antibodies per second.

work conclusively demonstrated that many infectious diseases are brought about by microorganisms storming the body's defenses (*Chapter* 1). More astonishing still, they established that disease-causing microbes could actually be separated, cultured, and manipulated as a way to protect people from infection.

Using his doctor's office as a laboratory and a microscope as his chief tool, Koch developed processes for isolating cultures of bacterial growth. His first major contribution came in 1876, when he pinpointed the organism that caused anthrax, a disease of hoofed animals that could decimate herds of sheep, cattle, and other livestock. In rapid order, scientists went on to identify the bacteria responsible for a range of other diseases, including diphtheria, typhoid fever, typhus, tetanus, and tuberculosis.

Koch's methods for identifying and growing bacteria catapulted disease research into a new era, but it took the genius of Pasteur—and a serendipitous error—to harness the extraordinary protective potential of germs. In the latter part of the 19th century, a cholera epidemic was wreaking havoc on the chicken industry in France. Desperate for a remedy, the country turned to Pasteur, who years earlier had become something of a national hero for his discovery that heating wine would prevent

spoilage, a process now known as pasteurization.

After two years of assiduously collecting and analyzing the feces of diseased chickens, Pasteur managed to isolate the guilty organism. Using Koch's method for growing culture media, he began producing cholera bacteria in strains so pure and thick that they quickly started to outgrow their nutrients. Pasteur found that he constantly had to transfer flourishing colonies of this cholera "broth" to new flasks to keep the organisms from poisoning themselves in their own waste products.

During the course of his investigation, Pasteur found that chickens fed even a few drops of the bacteria on a piece of bread inevitably died. But one day by mistake, he took an old culture that had been growing for weeks and fed it to a group of young, healthy chickens. To the scientist's surprise, the birds did not get sick. He purposefully fed old bacteria to another group of birds, with the same results. So he tried an experiment: Taking a vibrant new culture of cholera bacteria, he fed some to a different healthy group of chickens and the rest to the birds that had accidentally been exposed to the old

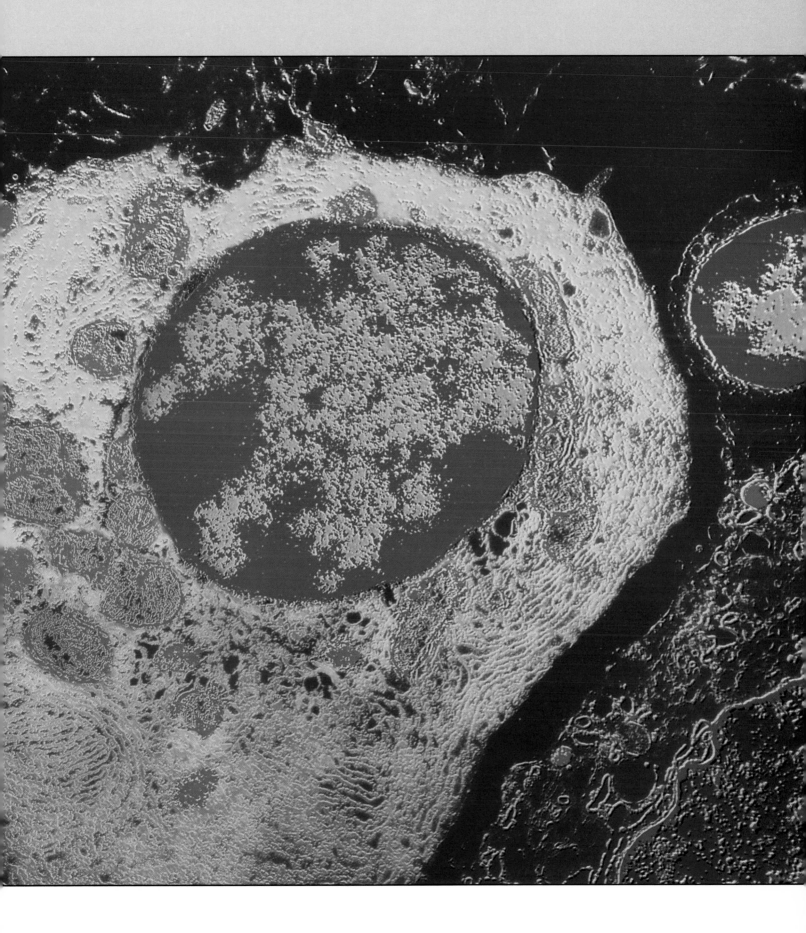

culture. Every one of these "healthy" chickens died. But all of the birds that had been fed the old, weakened bacteria survived.

Pasteur realized immediately that the weakened bacteria had somehow given the birds immunity from cholera. The implications were staggering. Perhaps, he reasoned, any disease-causing microbe could be rendered less potent by passing it through successive generations in the artificial conditions of the laboratory, then recruited to fight the very disease it once brought about.

Pasteur continued his experiments with anthrax, which was rapidly thinning the animal herds of France. Again borrowing techniques from Koch, the scientist isolated the organisms and grew them by the millions in culture dishes. This time, though, instead of weakening the bacteria, he killed them with phenol and injected the dead organisms into sheep. Result: None of the animals got sick. Just as weakened cholera bacteria had protected chickens, the killed anthrax organisms gave the sheep immunity from that disease. Before long, sheep and cows all over Europe were safe from the ravages of anthrax, thanks to Pasteur's vaccine.

But the French scientist's most stunning—and risky—breakthrough was yet to come. Turning his attention to rabies, Pasteur found that this of-

ten fatal disease of mammals was caused not by bacteria but by some mystery substance, which he knew was carried in the saliva of rabid animals. (Scientists today know what Pasteur did not: Rabies, like smallpox, is caused not by a bacterium but by a virus, an infinitesimally smaller microbe that is invisible under an ordinary microscope.) In time, Pasteur learned that he could immunize dogs against rabies by injecting the animals with bits of brain tissue removed from infected rabbits.

Before Pasteur had completed his investigation, however, a moment of truth arrived—on his doorstep. On July 5, 1885, a woman appeared unannounced at his laboratory in Alsace, accompanied by her nine-year-old son. The boy had been bitten 14 times by a dog that by all indications was rabid. Although Pasteur was not a doctor, he realized that the youngster could be dead within weeks, or as soon as the rabies infection had traveled from the nerve endings in the wounds to the brain. Risking prosecution for practicing medicine without a license—or imprisonment if his methods proved fatal—Pasteur decided to administer his new rabies vaccine in the hope of saving the boy's life.

Fortunately for both researcher and subject, the procedure worked; the boy survived the bites as well as the cure. Three months later Pasteur broke the news in a scientific paper, in which he declared that his vaccine had previously been tested on 50 dogs without a single failure. Alas, the great Pasteur was lying. Researchers who have since gone through his notebooks discovered that the French scientist had taken an extraordinary chance with the life of the child, injecting him with successively stronger doses of rabies virus.

As the notebooks revealed, Pasteur had been experimenting with this new technique on dogs, but as yet he had no evidence that it would work. In fact, the only animals he had successfully immunized so far had received the injections before they were subjected to the disease. Recalling the incident later, Pasteur admitted that he could not sleep the night before he gave the final injection. "The material I was using was so deadly, so undiluted," he wrote, "that it killed an unprotected rabbit in less than a day."

In today's medical environment, Pasteur's decision to experiment with the life of a child surely would have plunged the scientist into an ethical and legal quagmire. History might have regarded him in a harsher light had he failed. And yet, because he guessed correctly and succeeded, his image as a hero remains untarnished, and his rabies vaccine has come to be viewed not as madness but as brilliant science, a medical milestone. Pasteur's extensive findings about the body's microscopic enemies had provided scientists and physicians with a powerful new tool: By introducing altered or killed disease-causing agents into the body, they could help the natural defense mechanism fight back as never before.

Although Pasteur took advantage of the body's incredible capacity to arm itself, the eminent scientist could shed no light on the deeper mystery: How does one acquire this immunity? This fundamental question was soon to engage the minds of other scientists, who produced a flurry of promising discoveries and dazzling new theories. Almost immediately, though, these pathologists, immunologists, and bacteriologists aligned themselves with one of the two distinct

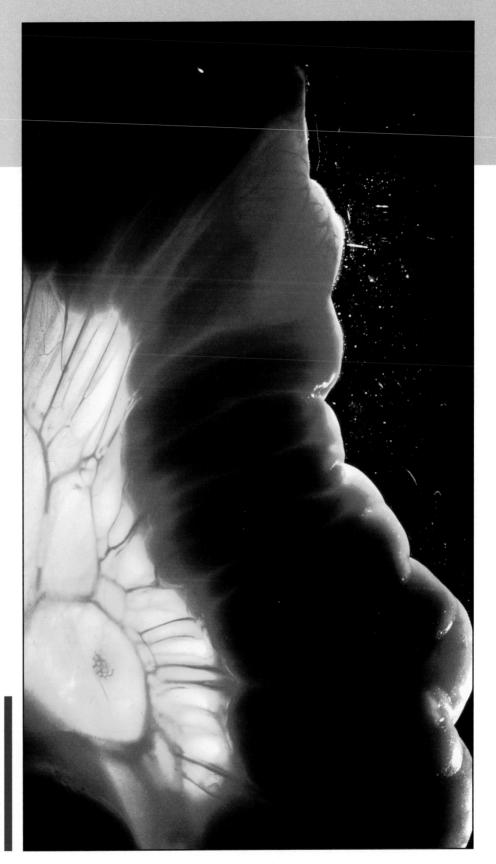

Seldom idle, lymph nodes such as this one from a human abdomen are frequent battlegrounds in the body's struggle against disease. Plasma cells and other forces of the immune system take position in these structures, ready to strike at bacteria, viruses, or other invaders. Swollen, aching lymph nodes signal a fierce encounter.

48

When Germs Get
Under the Skin

Although skin serves as a highly effective barrier against many types of invasions, breaks in the body's armor can allow harmful microbes or other antigens to pour into the underlying tissue. When this happens, the body mobilizes a defense called the inflammatory response. The classic symptoms of inflammation—redness, swelling, heat, and pain—are all signs that the invading forces are under attack.

As illustrated at right, among the immune system's inflammation strategies is the teaming of antigen-specific antibodies with complement, an intricate set of protein molecules so named because they complement the work of antibodies. An invader that penetrates the skin is greeted by an antibody, and the two lock together to create what is known as an antibody-antigen complex. This union attracts complement components, which latch onto the complex to actuate a series of molecular reactions. Factors loosed during this so-called complement cascade perform various functions, but their primary mission is to recruit voracious white blood cells called neutrophils from nearby capillaries. The neutrophils follow a trail established by complement back to the infection site and devour the invading antigens.

Most of the symptoms associated with the inflammatory response are by-products of this sophisticated recruitment process. For example, capillaries bringing in fresh supplies of blood dilate; as a result, the region becomes red and swollen. The capillaries also leak, allowing red blood cells, neutrophils, and other immune cells to flood the infected area. The buildup of pressure from blood rushing into the tissue produces heat and, along with chemicals released by immune cells, can cause pain—a signal that most likely will lead the individual to protect the area while the invasion is being neutralized.

When bacteria enter through a break in the skin, the body is prepared with custom-made antibodies—produced during a previous encounter—that lock onto the invaders. Nearby, a memory B cell of the same vintage awaits the chemical message that will cause it to differentiate into plasma cells and spawn a new wave of antibodies. As complement seeks out antibody-antigen complexes, blood-borne neutrophils and red blood cells pass through a capillary not far away (inset, bottom).

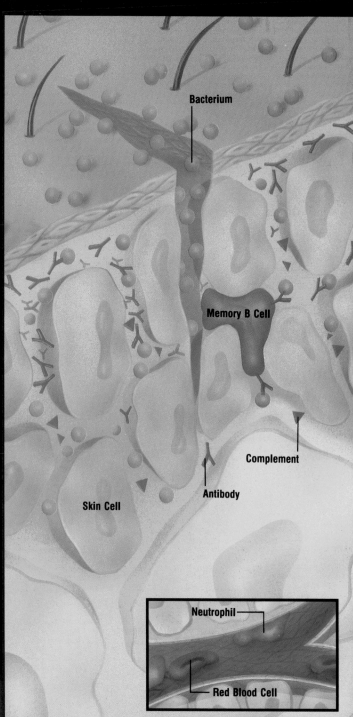

Bacterium

Memory B Cell

Complement

Antibody

Skin Cell

Neutrophil

Red Blood Cell

49

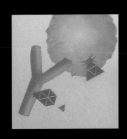

After binding to an antibody-antigen complex, complement begins to form protein fragments, some of which attach to antigens directly, either punching holes in the membrane wall *(left)* or marking them for annihilation by neutrophils. Others migrate toward the blood vessel *(below);* some of these fragments cause the capillary to expand, increasing blood flow and weakening the vessel wall *(inset, bottom).*

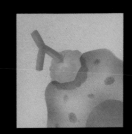

Responding to the chemical message, neutrophils squeeze between cells in the weakened capillary wall, which also allows red blood cells to escape, further inflaming the area. The neutrophils then follow the complement trail past skin cells to the infected region, where antibody-antigen complexes are located. A neutrophil destroys an antigen by engulfing it *(left)* and then injecting lethal chemicals. Macrophages will arrive later to consume any remaining debris.

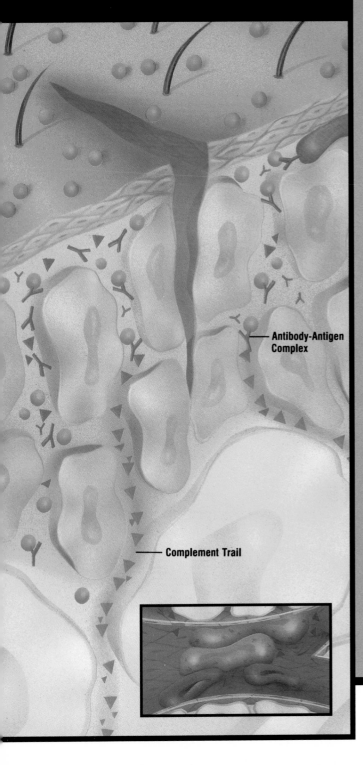

Antibody-Antigen Complex

Complement Trail

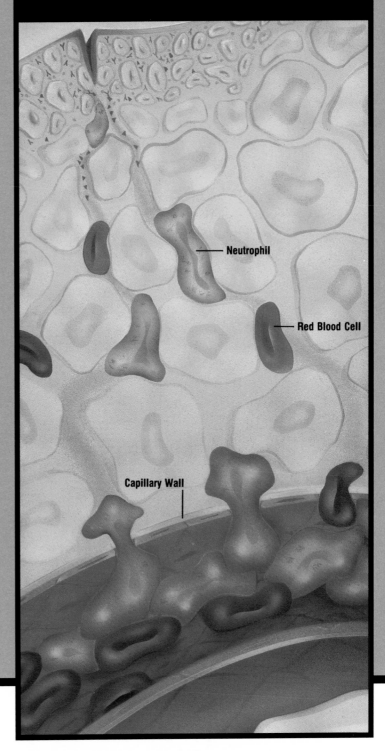

Neutrophil

Red Blood Cell

Capillary Wall

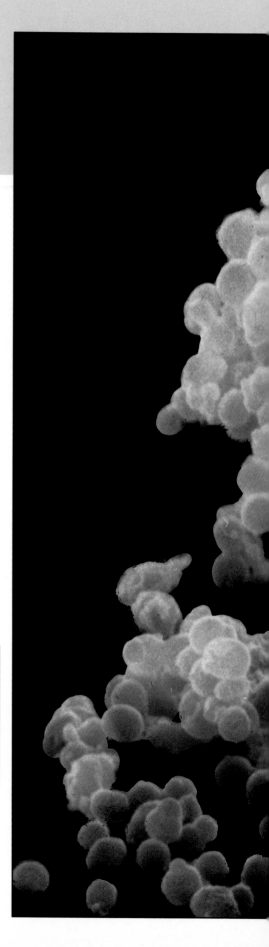

camps that were then debating the very nature of the immune system at its most fundamental level.

On the one side, of course, stood the cellularists, who, like Russian-born biologist Élie Metchnikoff, believed that immunity rested exclusively with the armies of scavenging, organism-gobbling white blood cells called phagocytes. On the other side, Robert Koch and his followers were asserting with equal vehemence that the task of immobilizing and destroying germs was carried out not by cells but by toxic substances borne by the blood and other bodily fluids. By 1890 the balance seemed to have tipped heavily in favor of this latter faction, the so-called humoralists. That year, news had emerged from the University of Berlin that Emil von Behring and Japanese bacteriologist Shibasaburo Kitasato had discovered disease-fighting "antitoxins" in blood serum—the legions of aggressive little defenders that would later become known as antibodies.

While the cellularists and humoralists continued their intellectual warfare, each side refusing to relent, one scientist stepped forward in 1898 with an audacious theory that seemed to bridge the two camps, although it was unprovable with the scientific tools of the period. German chemist Paul Ehrlich was trying to determine the specific concentration of antibodies in

blood serum it takes to neutralize diphtheria toxin. Observations he made in the course of his work at the Institute of Experimental Research in Frankfurt led him to a notion about the architecture of white blood cells.

Clinging to the surfaces of these cells, Ehrlich suggested, was a variety of knoblike appendages, which he called side chains. Should such a cell encounter an invading substance, his theory went, one of these side chains would fit into a corresponding slot on the foreigner's surface, and the two would snap together like pieces of a jigsaw puzzle. Immediately, the cell would respond by manufacturing huge numbers of similar side chains, which would then break free and spill out into the blood to function as circulating antibodies. The chemist even sketched out his vision of the phenomenon, showing increasing numbers of fish-shaped invaders clamping

Reacting to an allergy-causing substance on its surface, a tissue cell releases histamine (yellow) and other chemicals (blue) that help regulate the immune system. Histamine dilates blood vessels, bringing more defenders to the site, and causes the sneezing and watery eyes typical of an allergic reaction.

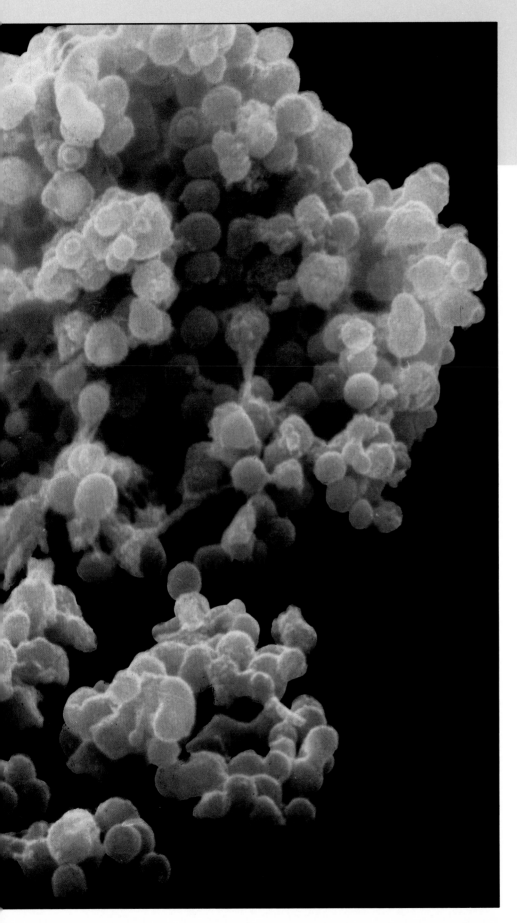

onto a cell's protruding receptors. Ehrlich's primitive cartoon drawings vexed his colleagues. For example, Belgian bacteriologist Jules Bordet, who a few years earlier had spelled out the intricacies of how antibodies and the complex molecules known as complement worked together in the immune response, dismissed Ehrlich's depictions as "puerile."

As scientists have since determined, however, all three of these views were accurate, at least to some degree. Metchnikoff's phagocytes do indeed defend the body from foreign invasion, some staking out permanent posts in the spleen and liver, while others circulate throughout the body, migrating into such organs as the lungs, kidneys, and brain to destroy invading organisms. The humoralists' assertion that substances in the blood fight disease-causing organisms has also been borne out time and again by research into antibodies, which sometimes coat foreign particles, making clumps that form conspicuous targets for gluttonous phagocytes. And Ehrlich's imaginative renderings of cells latching onto enemy targets, if wrong in some important details, were so close to being correct that immunologists today still

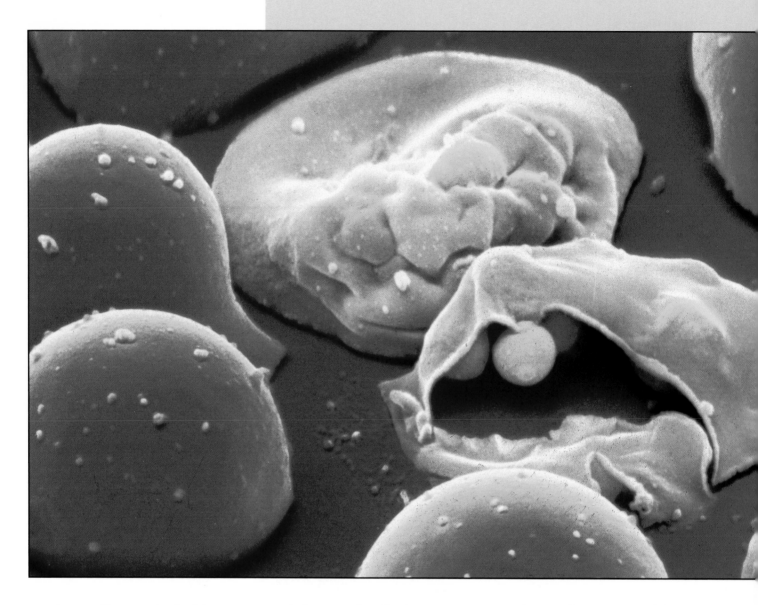

use them to illustrate the body's acquired immune reaction.

By the turn of the 20th century, a rudimentary understanding of the mechanisms of immunity was starting to take shape, but scientists remained largely in the dark about how the body could build up, or acquire, such formidable defenses. Some of the most illuminating early insights came from the laboratory of Karl Landsteiner, an Austrian-born immunologist who spent more than three decades demonstrating how precisely attuned antibodies are to invaders. In tests with rabbits mostly at the Rockefeller Institute for Medical Research in New York, Landsteiner discovered that every substance he introduced into an animal induced the production of highly specific antibodies. That is, the immune system appeared capable of manufacturing an unlimited range of antibodies to combat any foreign material thrown at it—whether naturally occurring or conjured in a test tube.

The notion that antibody formation was determined by the nature of the intruder contrasted sharply with Ehrlich's side-chain theory, which assumed that each cell was designed with a sufficient variety of receptors, or antibodies, to accommodate all comers. A number of ideas arose to take its place, however, including a proposal in the 1930s by American chemist Linus Pauling.

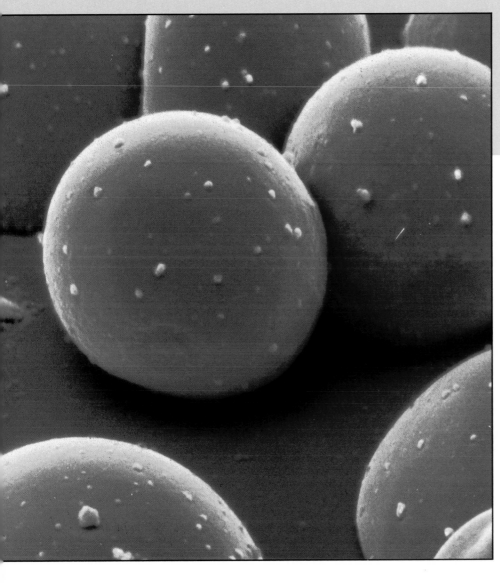

disease-causing agent so much stronger after the first encounter? The picture came into sharper focus in 1957, when Macfarlane Burnet—the Australian virologist whose insights a decade earlier helped prove that the body's tolerance to "foreign" cells could be modified—postulated that cells in the immune system can recognize an infinite number of microbes even before the combatants meet.

Picking up essentially where Ehrlich left off, Burnet proposed that some of the immune system's specialized cells have on their outer membranes almost half a million receptors, or specific arrangements of protein molecules that recall the knoblike protuberances on Ehrlich's model. Unlike Ehrlich, however, Burnet suggested that each cell displays identical receptors—many locks that match the keys of only one type of antigen. According to Burnet's "clonal selection theory," when a receptor, or lock, binds to an antigen with the proper key, the cell begins to enlarge and divide at a dizzying pace, turning itself into a mass-production factory for clones (genetically identical reproductions) of that particular kind of cell. These clones, called plasma cells, in turn discharge swarms of customized antibodies into

By this time, scientists had learned that antibodies are immunoglobulins, or globular proteins, so named because their amino acid chains bend into roughly spherical shapes that can wrap around a disease-causing substance, or antigen. In this way, antibodies can "read" the intruder's surface—the only part that matters in triggering a response. (The body mistakes dead rabies for live rabies, for example, because the germs' outer membranes are identical.) In his "template theory" of antibody formation, Pauling hypothesized that an antibody gained specificity just by the shape it assumed as it folded around an antigen. But even Pauling's theory left many questions unanswered. What, for example, could explain the extraordinary mass production of "correct" antibodies after an antigen has been pegged? And why is the body's antibody reaction to a the bloodstream. Most plasma cells die after a few days, but others live on as so-called memory cells, which continue manufacturing that one kind of antibody long after the initial invasion has subsided.

Serving as the backbone of this elaborate defense network are the white blood cells that, when alerted to danger, metamorphose into antibody-producing plasma cells. These essential components of the immune system, called B lymphocytes, or B cells, originate in red bone marrow, the spongy tissue at the core of larger bones. Since the late 1950s, scientists have learned to stimulate B cells to make certain kinds of antibodies. When a doctor gives an infant its first dose of diphtheria, pertussis, and tetanus vaccine, for example, the shot stimulates the child's B cells to produce so-called immunoglobulin M (IgM) antibodies, which are very effective at binding to many kinds of bacteria. In recent years researchers also have learned that some degree of immunity can be transferred from one person to another—or from an animal to a human—by injections of blood serum rich in specific kinds of antibodies. This so-called passive immunity typically lasts only a few weeks or months, but it can afford useful protection from, say, snakebites or diseases such as botulism or tetanus. In some cases, however, the introduc-

tion of foreign antibodies can provoke a strong, even fatal, reaction from the recipient's own immune system.

Clonal selection was a major breakthrough, but it left some fundamental issues for later researchers to ponder. One of the biggest remaining conundrums about acquired immunity was the puzzle of recognition—that is, how do B cells distinguish foreign substances from cells and tissues of their human or animal "host"? An early clue was unearthed three decades ago, with the discovery that B cells are not alone in the fight against foreign aggression. In 1962, Jacques Miller, a young cancer investigator at the Chester Beatty Research Institute in London, was trying to determine the function of the thymus, a double-lobed gland, common to most vertebrates, that in humans is located behind the breastbone. The thymus withers after puberty and can be removed from adult animals or humans with no apparent effect. In an experiment, Miller carefully extracted the thymuses from newborn mice, then monitored the creatures' progress. Result: The mice survived, but they developed into runts with small numbers of lymphocytes, a deficiency that severely hindered the animals' ability

to mount effective immune responses. In follow-up studies that same year, Oxford University researchers James L. Gowans and Douglas McGregor injected lymphocytes into mice whose thymuses had been destroyed or weakened by radiation. The animals quickly recovered their ability to fight infections, offering dramatic evidence of the crucial role lymphocytes play in warding off disease.

These and other experiments led the way to the realization that not all lymphocytes are created equal. All of these specialized white blood cells begin life in the bone marrow, and those destined to become B cells remain there until fully developed. Afterward, mature B cells ship out to stations in the body's lymph nodes to guard against attacks and release antibodies into the bloodstream. Other lymphocytes, however, leave the bone marrow before maturity and migrate to exclusive cell training grounds in the thymus, where each cell learns to recognize a specific antigen. Through some still-unknown mechanism in the thymus, cells are also taught to identify the molecules, known as major histocompatibility complex (MHC) proteins, that mark the membranes of host cells like flags of biological nationality.

Cells in training that are prone to attack "friendly" cells are weeded out, as are those that have trouble

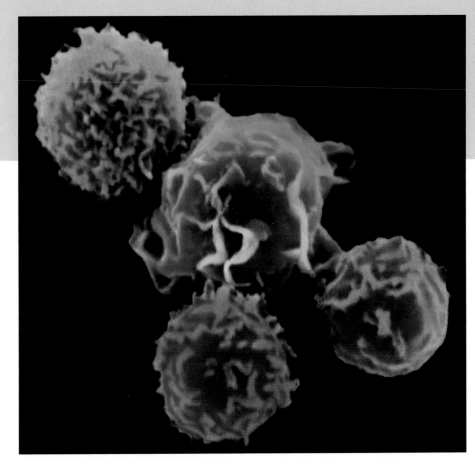

distinguishing intruders. Indeed, as many as 99 percent of these thymus-educated cells will die—perhaps, as microbiologist Mark Davis of Stanford University in Palo Alto, California, put it, because the body selects only "those with the sharpest powers of recognition." Surviving T cells, so named for the gland where they are schooled, become the chief regulators of the immune system.

There are several distinct classes of T cells, all identical in appearance but distinguished by function. Helper T cells do not go into combat themselves but, as their name implies, as-

sist those cells that do. Some scientists, in fact, regard helper T cells as the "master switch" of the immune system. Using protein receptors similar to those on the surface of B cells, helper T cells detect the presence of specific antigens. Then, through various secretions, they summon reinforcements, instruct B cells to start making antibody-producing plasma cells, and foster the production of cytotoxic, or killer, T cells. These aggressive executioners of the immune system largely confine their attacks to body cells that have become infected with viruses. They bind to a target cell, and, rather than engulfing it as a phagocyte would, they shoot it full of holes using molecules of a lethal protein. Infected cells punctured in this

fashion leak and die, effectively destroying the virus before it has a chance to spread.

Another group of related lymphocytes are the natural killer (NK) cells. Specialists in battling cancerous cells, NK cells wander like lone wolves in the immune system, attacking antigens whether they recognize them or not. Some scientists also argue for the existence of yet another group, the so-called suppressor T cells, which act as the system's peacemakers, calling off the immune response after an invasion has been squelched.

Revelations about T cells opened yet another window on the acquired immune system, providing glimpses of a complex regulatory subsystem that tells the disease-fighting machinery when to go into action. For years, immunologists had assumed that the introduction of foreign particles into the body was the sole stimulus for activating the immune system. In recent years, scientists have discovered that, like most other systems in the body, the immune reaction is orchestrated by precisely timed secretions of specialized chemicals.

The first evidence of such a chemical-messenger system came to light with the discovery in 1957 of a

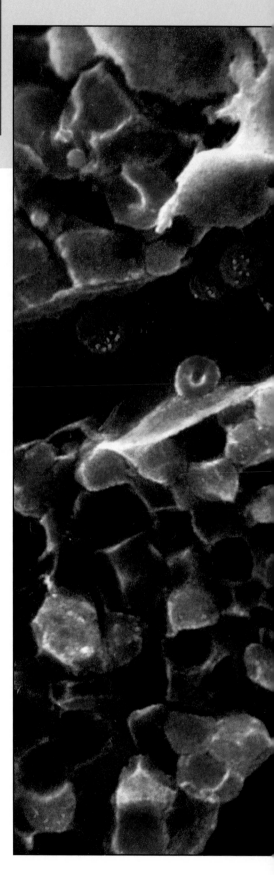

Immature red and white blood cells *(tinted red and blue)* cluster in the bone marrow where they were produced. In cases of severe blood loss, white cells that developed into memory cells would retreat to the marrow, preserving the immune system's ability to repel new onslaughts of invaders met in the past.

substance called interferon, believed to be one of the body's main defenses against viruses. Under attack by viral invaders, most cells release interferon, which quickly alerts other cells in the vicinity of an enemy invasion. No one knows exactly how interferon works, but the chemical seems to stimulate cells to produce a protein that, in effect, scrambles a virus's genetic instructions, making it impossible for the intruder to replicate.

Experiments conducted between 1978 and 1983 by Dartmouth University microbiologist Kendall A. Smith established that interferon is not the only chemical that plays a role in activating the immune system against invaders. In fact, Smith postulated that once a foreign substance has penetrated the body's defenses, a complex regulatory chemical network takes full control of the immune system. As he described the process, invaders are met and consumed by large scavenger phagocytes called macrophages, which display portions of their vanquished foes' molecules on their own membranes like captured enemy flags. Most T cells circulating through the bloodstream ignore these flags, but those that have been trained to recognize enemy colors are stirred to action. Just as B cells become superfactories for antibodies during an attack, these activated helper T cells start producing quanti-

ties of a hormone called interleukin-2 (IL-2), which in turn promotes the massive proliferation of still more helper T cells. IL-2 also helps stimulate the transformation of B cells into plasma cells, thereby triggering the release of antibodies.

As a constant stream of discoveries changes the face of immunology, each breakthrough adds one more piece to the acquired-immunity puzzle. Yet some of today's most startling revelations are echoes of lessons not learned in the past. As often happens in science, some notions are advanced before researchers have the tools to analyze and exploit them. Paul Ehrlich's theory of antibody production is such a notion, as is his related—and even bolder—concept of, in effect, antiantibodies.

Ehrlich speculated that the binding of an antibody with a foreign invader might trigger the production of another substance, an antigen of some sort that provokes a kind of counterattack from the immune system. In other words, the body might dispatch antibodies to its own antibodies. Like system executioners, these squads of cleanup proteins would, in Ehrlich's view, prevent the immune system

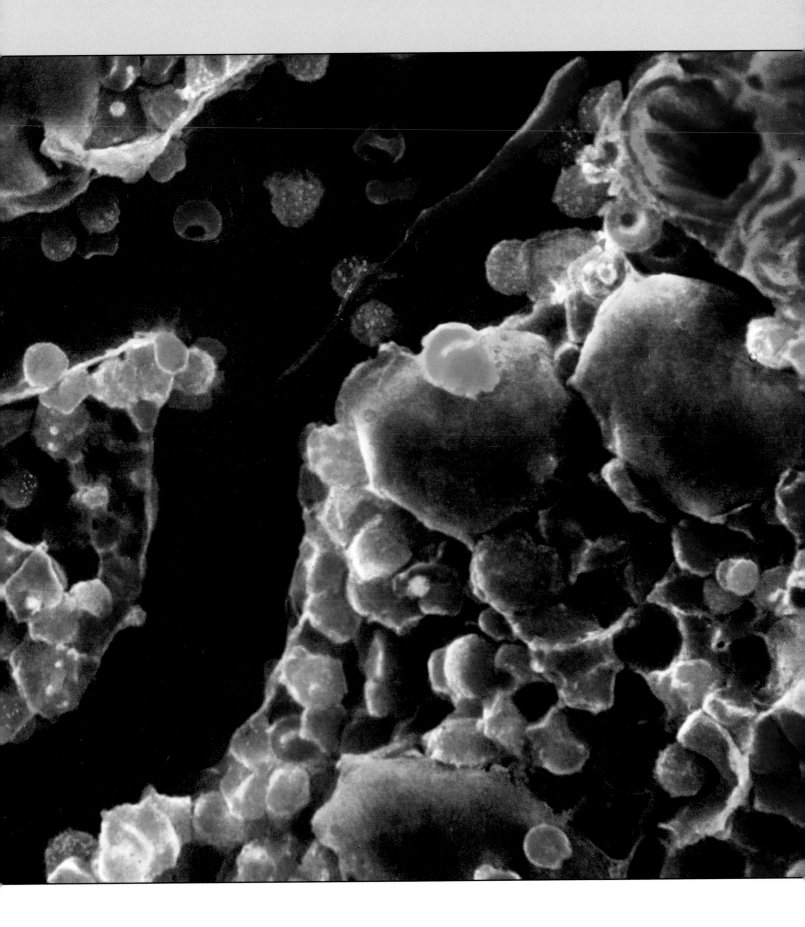

from spinning out of control and attacking the body indiscriminately.

Modern-day scientists have found that Ehrlich's theories about antiantibodies, like his theory of molecular side chains, may well have been right on the mark. Experiments with animals have shown that the body does produce some kind of antibody-fighting substance, perhaps as a way to suppress the immune reaction once the threat has passed. The first to put together a comprehensive theory of what might be taking place was Danish immunologist Niels Kaj Jerne, who proposed in 1974 that a modest production of antiantibodies was the normal state of affairs in the body rather than the exception—a routine function of a self-regulating mechanism. In his "network theory," Jerne put forth the notion that antibodies sent to fight intruders end up as targets themselves. He proposed that the body fires off antiantibodies in waves of decreasing intensity until the process slows to a halt.

Most immunologists today have come to accept Jerne's theory, which could have dramatic implications for researchers hoping to tap the potential of acquired immunity. One day, for example, doctors may be able to treat allergic reactions to, say, ragweed pollen with injections of antiantibodies to immunoglobulin E, or IgE, the antibody specifically geared

to fight ragweed. When IgE binds with ragweed pollen on the surface of some tissue cells, these cells start churning out histamine, a chemical that, among other things, increases secretion by mucous glands in the nose and lungs. The familiar symptoms—hives, hay fever, asthma—signal a massive mobilization of the immune system. In the future, though, it may be possible to suppress these unpleasant side effects by sending in a special unit of terminator antibodies that are trained to hunt down and destroy only those immune system antibodies targeting ragweed pollen.

Another promising use of antiantibodies—a technique that fools the immune system with a look-alike antigen—may be just around the corner. Researchers have found that some antiantibodies carry on their surface the same molecular flags as the antigens that elicited the immune response. Because these flags are what really matters to the system's defenders, introduction of such antiantibodies into the body can trigger an immune response similar to that caused by an injection of a live or killed microbe. A number of researchers have begun using this technique in an attempt to immunize animals against

viruses. And at the Southwest Foundation for Biomedical Research in San Antonio, Texas, scientists are investigating the possible use of antiantibodies as a treatment for melanomas, or malignant skin tumors, in people. The beauty of this method is that it can reduce risk: With live-virus vaccinations, for example, there is always a chance the procedure will backfire, triggering instead the development of the full-blown disease.

Since Edward Jenner's bold experiment with smallpox some two centuries ago, vaccinations for diseases of all types have saved untold millions of lives. But vaccines do have their drawbacks, and experts continue to argue their merits. For example, a debate rages over polio vaccines. Scandinavian countries immunize their populations with the killed-virus vaccine devised by Jonas Salk in the mid-1950s, while the United States uses the live, weakened version developed five years later by Albert Sabin. The advantage of the live vaccine is that, once inside the body, it reproduces profusely, forcing the immune system to develop a strong, often lifelong immunity. Killed viruses, on the other hand, may provide lasting immunity, but periodic booster shots are often required to "remind" the body of its immunization. The live virus, however, has a troublesome disadvantage: Once the weak-

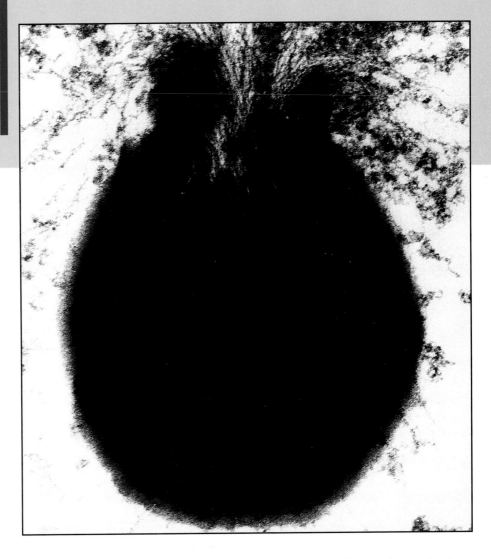

Weakened by an experimental antibiotic, a *Staphylococcus aureus* bacterium, which can cause pneumonia and bone disease, explodes in a cascade of cytoplasm. Researchers once regarded antibiotics as wonder drugs—until they discovered that some bacteria fight back, building up resistance of their own and producing generations of drug-resistant germs.

ened germ is introduced into a patient, doctors have no way of controlling its possibly harmful mutations.

As hindsight makes clear, many of the successes of the past 200 years in the field of immunology have come at great expense. Even the most profound breakthroughs can bring on dire and unexpected complications. The discovery of penicillin in 1928 is a case in point. In a wave of euphoria about the cure-all properties of antibiotics, or germ-killing drugs, American pharmaceutical companies began the painstaking process of researching and developing penicillin. By 1942, enough of the drug had been produced to treat but a single patient. A year later, however, 100 patients had been treated, and by the time of D-day in 1944, enough penicillin was on hand to treat all the British and American troops seriously injured in the Allied invasion of Europe.

But high hopes for this perceived wonder drug were quickly dampened. Having harnessed the adaptability of the body's immune system to fight disease through vaccinations, scientists had failed to take into account the remarkable ability of bacteria to fight back. For example, many strains of staphylococci, or staph, and gonor-

rhea microorganisms rapidly became resistant to penicillin, producing an enzyme, penicillinase, that rendered the antibiotic inactive. Hospitals became breeding grounds for penicillin-resistant germs; newborns and patients with burns or operative wounds became particularly susceptible to staph infections. At one London hospital, for example, bacteriologists found that 12.5 percent of staphylococci cultured from patients' respiratory tracts were resistant to penicillin in 1946, 38 percent in 1947, and 59 percent in 1948. Five years later, staph bacteria in 73 percent of the

patients at one hospital in Finland were highly resistant to the drug.

To complicate matters, growing supplies and falling prices contributed to penicillin's overuse. And so did the illusion of complete safety. Unlike vaccinations, which allow the body to do what it would do naturally—letting the acquired immune system run the show—penicillin conferred no immunity. If anything, the drug blinded the immune system to danger. Over time, doctors learned to refrain from using the antibiotic when it was not needed, to avoid excessive doses, and to always ask patients about past allergic reactions before administering the drug. Thanks to such precautions, penicillin and other antibiotics have again in recent years become effective agents in the war against disease—but not without a sobering lesson on the folly of "wonder drugs."

The acquired immune system, however adaptable and sophisticated it may be, is hardly fail-safe. Even at its best it remains vulnerable to a host of deadly and resourceful enemies. Some viruses—most notably HIV, the culprit behind acquired immunodeficiency syndrome (AIDS)—assault the immune system itself, crippling the body's defenses by destroying the helper T cells that sound the alarm and are vital for an effective immune response. Others, such as the herpesvirus, hide inside cells until the body lowers its defenses, then undergo replicating frenzies that lead to painful lesions on the skin and mucous membranes. A number of viruses camouflage themselves by raising different protein flags on their membranes virtually at random, in effect making every assault a new learning experience for the immune system. The quick-change abilities of influenza viruses, for example, keep the system guessing and account for annual winter outbreaks of the flu.

No attack, however, is so devastating as one from within. Despite its elaborate system of checks and balances, sometimes the body's defensive machinery goes horribly awry, turning on the very cells and tissues it is designed to protect. Such is the nightmare of autoimmunity, a range of often fatal diseases in which the body's enemy is the body itself. Until recently, scientists were convinced that such immunological destruction was impossible, so complete was their faith in the body's capacity for self-regulation. That they were mistaken is as clear as the challenge for scientists pushing forward into new frontiers of immunology.

THE CALL TO ARMS

Our ability to fight infection is based on the body's skill at distinguishing self from nonself. Almost every cell in the body has distinctive molecules—MHC-I and MHC-II, for example—that identify it as self; generally, the immune system attacks as foreign all substances with different markers. Such provoking agents, known as antigens, include viruses, bacteria, parasites, and fungi.

An infectious agent introduced to the body first encounters the nonspecific, or innate, immune response involving mechanisms that work against a broad range of invaders. If this defense proves insufficient, the specific, or acquired, immune response begins, with weapons tailored to battle the particular microorganism. The acquired immune response also includes the creation of special "memory" cells that ensure an even more vigorous reaction to subsequent invasions by the same pathogen.

The scenario on the following pages depicts an immune response to an infection by influenza virus, lasting one to two weeks. The primary site is the trachea (*right*), an airway lined with epithelial cells and surrounded by connective tissue and an outer layer of cartilage. Counterattacking immune cells arrive via blood vessels.

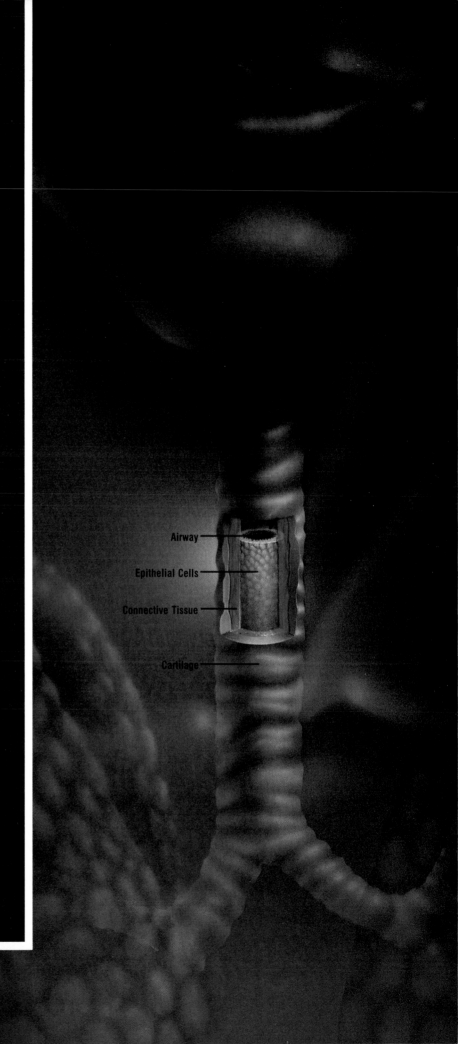

Airway

Epithelial Cells

Connective Tissue

Cartilage

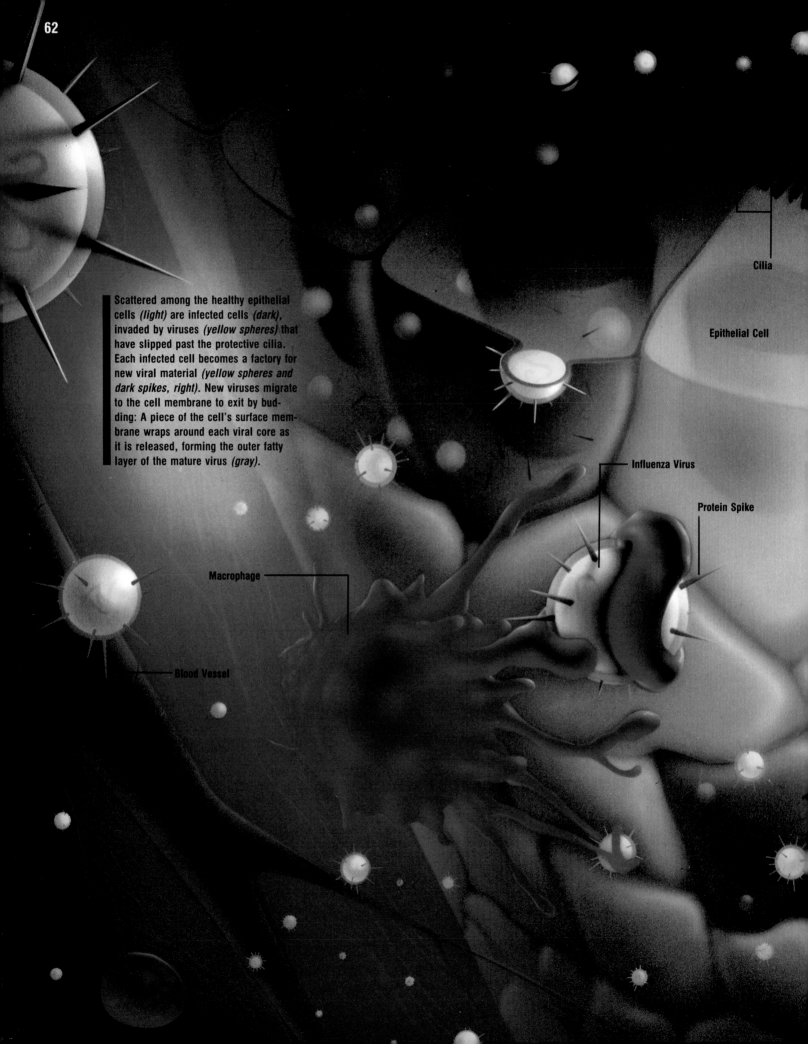

Scattered among the healthy epithelial cells *(light)* are infected cells *(dark)*, invaded by viruses *(yellow spheres)* that have slipped past the protective cilia. Each infected cell becomes a factory for new viral material *(yellow spheres and dark spikes, right)*. New viruses migrate to the cell membrane to exit by budding: A piece of the cell's surface membrane wraps around each viral core as it is released, forming the outer fatty layer of the mature virus *(gray)*.

Cilia

Epithelial Cell

Influenza Virus

Protein Spike

Macrophage

Blood Vessel

GENERAL ALERT

Penetration of the body's first line of defense (*pages* 16-19) sets the immune response in motion. With an influenza infection, this happens when viruses in the trachea evade the cilia, hairlike projections from the epithelium that trap most foreign particles. Protein spikes on the viruses give them an ingrained affinity for the epithelial cells lining the airway.

The invaders, which cannot replicate themselves independently, work their way into the epithelium and hijack the cellular machinery to churn out new viruses. Thus, to eliminate the infection, the immune system must not only wipe out the viruses but get rid of infected host cells as well.

The first nonspecific immune activity comes from the infected epithelial cells, which release interferon (*not shown*), one of a class of chemical messengers called cytokines. Interferon signals healthy cells to protect themselves against infection by producing proteins that inhibit viral activity.

The body's immune reaction continues with the arrival of macrophages, free-ranging white blood cells that swallow up any nonself matter they encounter. The macrophages set the stage for the specific response by processing viruses into a form that can be recognized by immune cells targeting this particular antigen.

The macrophages also release cytokines that signal the hypothalamus to raise the body's temperature. The resulting fever inhibits viral activity. For the flu victim, this first symptom of illness is often accompanied by a sore throat, caused by swelling as the virus destroys epithelial cells.

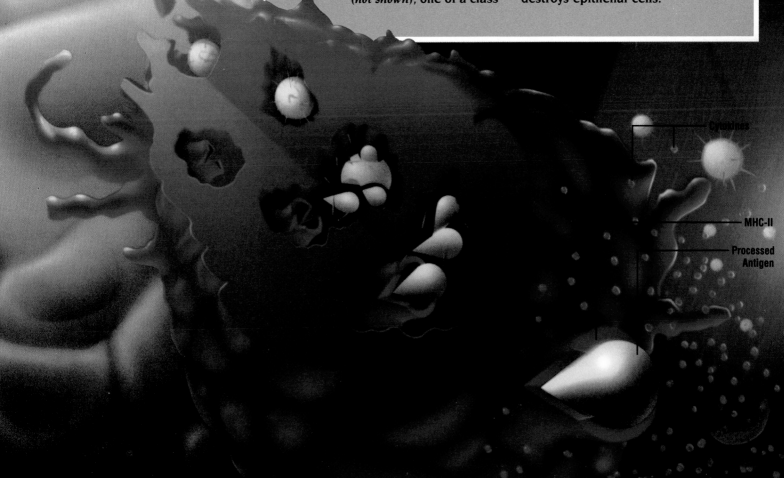

A macrophage (*left*) snares an attacker by extending a pseudopod. Another macrophage (*below*) begins to process a captured virus by engulfing it in a vesicle. As chemical reactions break the virus apart, the vesicle joins another vesicle carrying an MHC-II self-marker molecule. A fragment of the processed virus binds with MHC-II, and the resulting complex moves to the surface of the macrophage. At this time the macrophage releases cytokines (*blue dots*).

Cytokines

MHC-II

Processed Antigen

CALLING UP REINFORCEMENTS

The specific immune response begins in earnest with the recruitment of a cellular army of lymphocytes that can recognize and attack the invader. The main combatants will be B cells and cytotoxic T cells (also known as killer T cells), but the key role falls to another lymphocyte, the helper T cell, which signals other cells to multiply and launch the attack.

Only a few of the cells that circulate through the lymphatic system are tailored to respond to the flu virus (*pages 32-35*). To play its part in the attack, each of these cells must receive two different types of stimuli. The cell must first interact with its specific antigen and then receive signals from cytokines that prompt it to proliferate and differentiate. When both of these conditions are met, the immune cell is said to be activated.

When a helper T cell encounters and binds to the self-marker-antigen complex on the surface of a macrophage, a cascade of chemical events begins. Cytokines from the macrophage prompt the helper T cell to release its own cytokines, which in turn stimulate it and other T cells to proliferate. The resulting legion of T cells is custom-made to recognize and fight the specific foreign agent.

The flood of cytokines from an activated helper T cell also activates other lymphocytes. A B cell, for example, which finds the first key to activation when it binds to a free-floating virus, responds to the helper T cell's cytokines by proliferating and differentiating into memory B cells and antibody-producing plasma cells.

A helper T cell *(right)* binds to the MHC-II-antigen complex on the macrophage. Cytokines from the macrophage and helper T cell complete the signal that causes the helper T cell to multiply *(below)*. The result is a colony of antigen-specific helper T cells and memory T cells. The helper T cell also releases cytokines to activate a killer T cell *(below)* and B cells *(far right)*, both specific to this viral antigen.

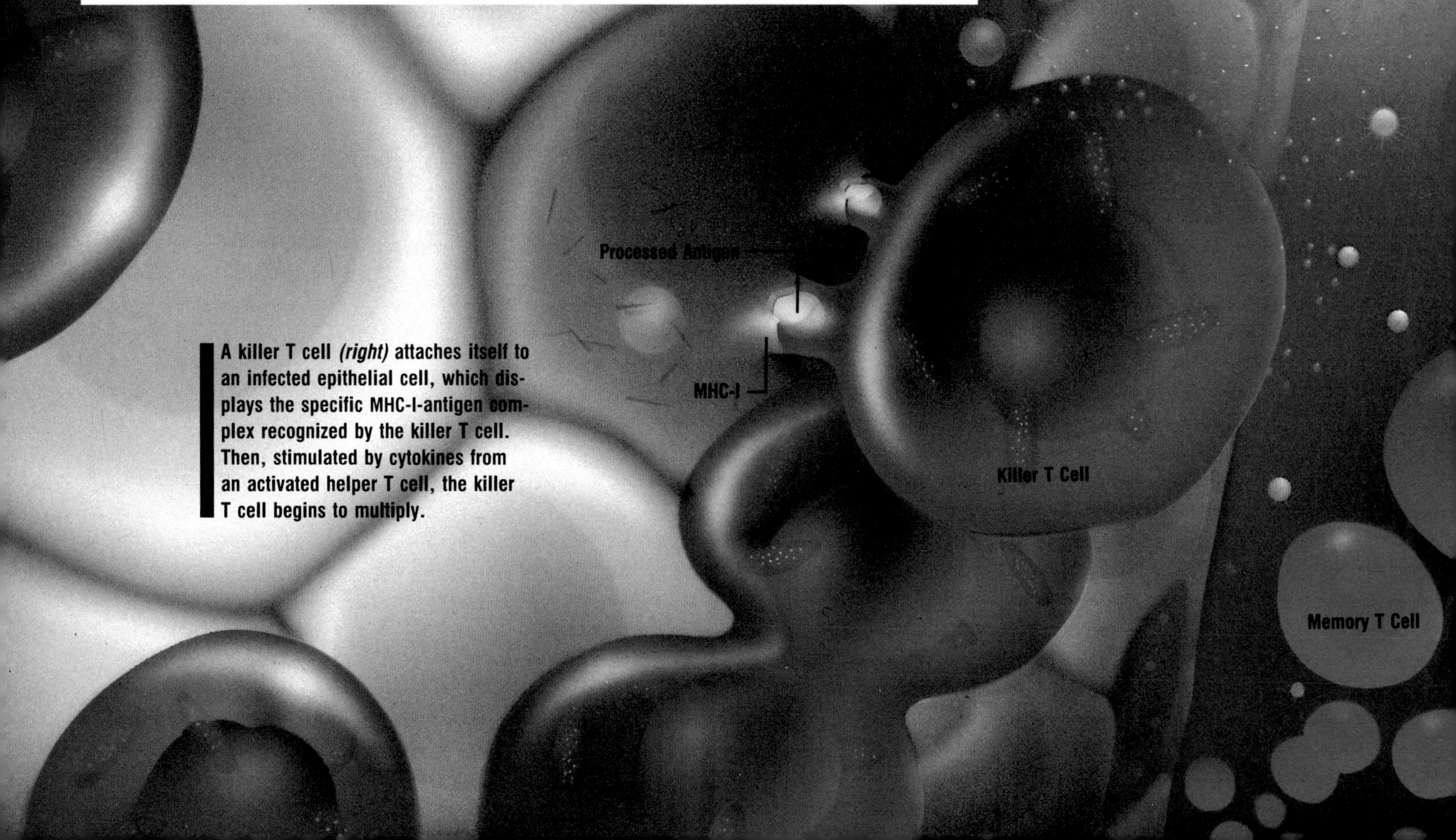

Processed Antigen

MHC-I

Killer T Cell

A killer T cell *(right)* attaches itself to an infected epithelial cell, which displays the specific MHC-I-antigen complex recognized by the killer T cell. Then, stimulated by cytokines from an activated helper T cell, the killer T cell begins to multiply.

Memory T Cell

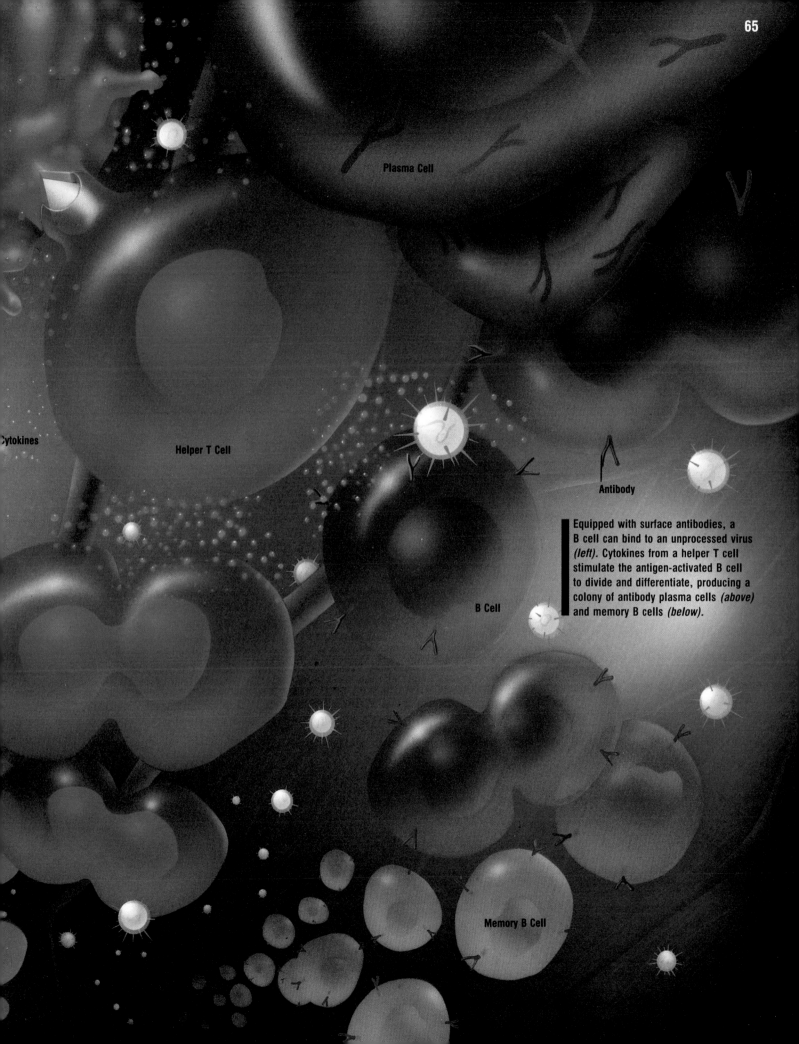

Plasma Cell

Cytokines

Helper T Cell

Antibody

B Cell

Equipped with surface antibodies, a B cell can bind to an unprocessed virus *(left)*. Cytokines from a helper T cell stimulate the antigen-activated B cell to divide and differentiate, producing a colony of antibody plasma cells *(above)* and memory B cells *(below)*.

Memory B Cell

ATTACK

Now activated specifically against the infecting virus, the hordes of immune cells conduct a two-pronged campaign. One prong, the cell-mediated response, destroys the infected cells that produce copies of the invader; the so-called humoral response combats free-floating viruses.

In the cell-mediated response, killer T cells bind to the MHC-I-antigen complex on cells that are producing copies of the virus. There they release proteins called perforins, which cause pores to form in the target cell's outer membrane, admitting other toxic substances that eventually kill the cell. The killer T cells are unharmed by perforins and can detach and move on to target other infected cells.

In the humoral response, plasma cells secrete antibodies that travel to the bloodstream and circulate throughout the body. The antibodies bind to free-floating viruses, disarming them and tagging them for disposal by cleanup macrophages. Some of these antibody-virus complexes also activate so-called complement proteins (*page* 21); circulating in the blood, the complement proteins trigger other aspects of the immune response, including the release of histamine to cause inflammation.

Histamine enhances the permeability of the blood vessels, increasing circulation and bringing more immune cells to the battle site. The redness, warmth, and swelling of the inflammation contribute to the discomfort of the flu sufferer. The full effects of the battle within include not only a sore throat but also a runny nose, sneezing, coughing, and swollen glands.

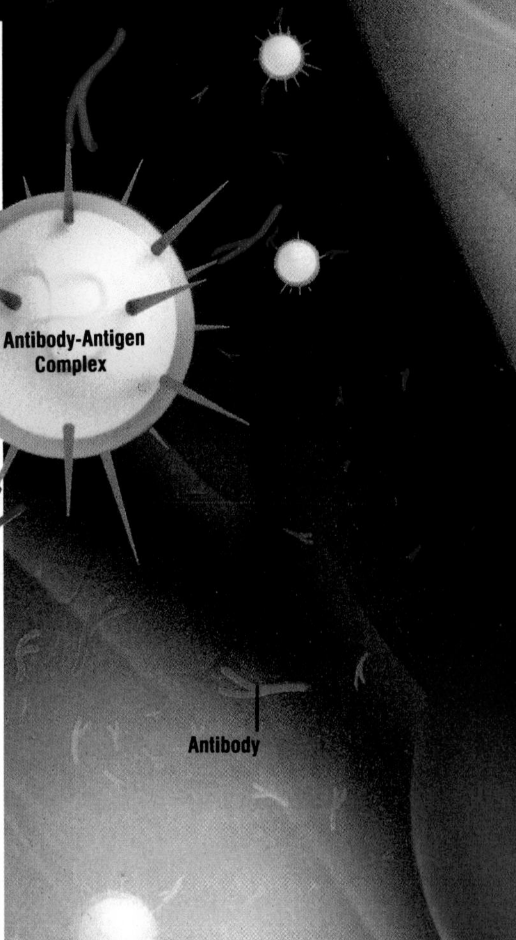

Antibody-Antigen Complex

Antibody

Plasma cells *(below)* begin producing antibodies *(red Y-shaped particles)* at the rate of 2,000 per second. The antibodies bind to free-floating viruses *(above)*, preventing them from attaching to uninfected epithelial cells and marking them as targets for macrophages soon to arrive on the scene.

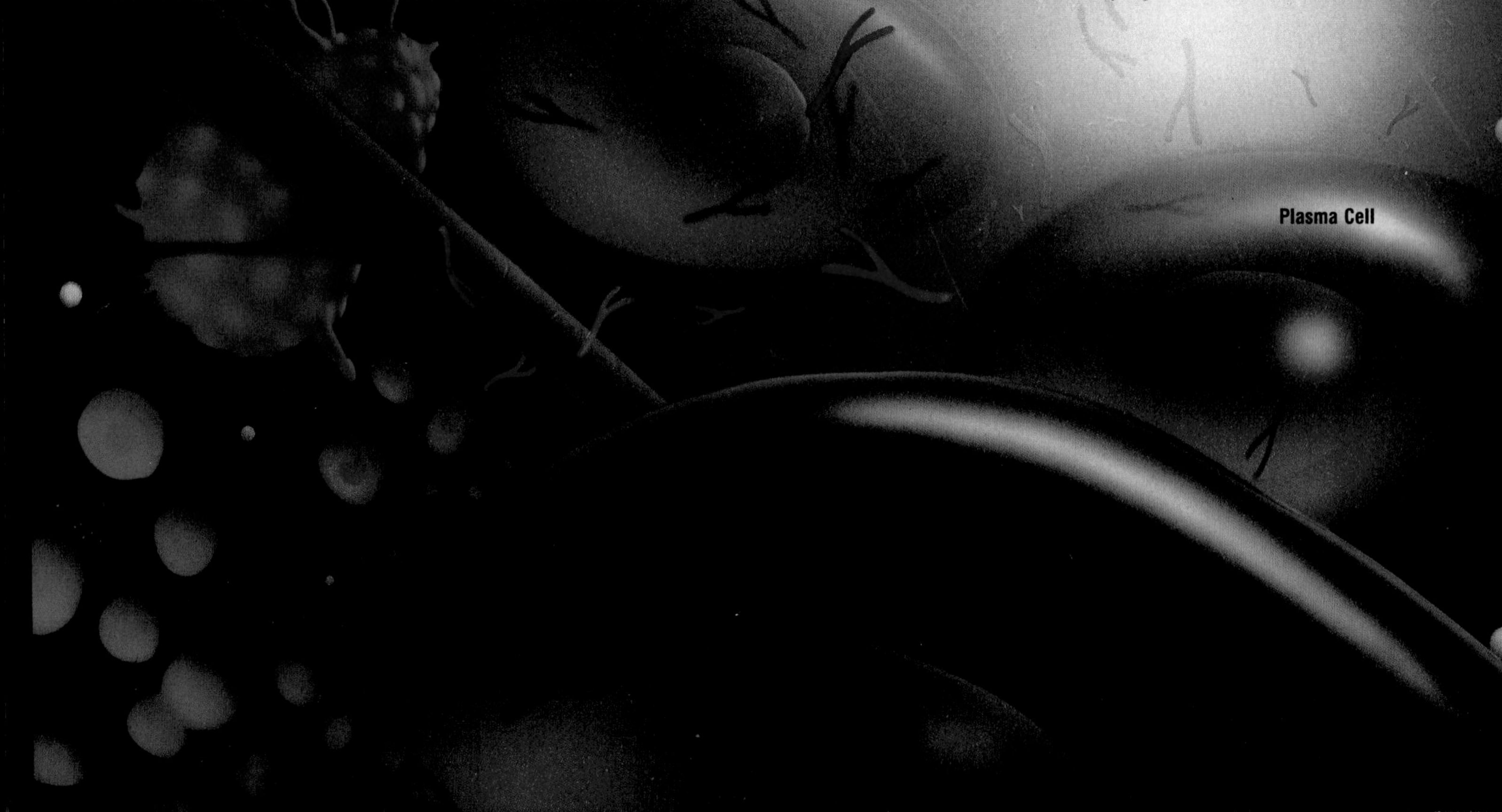

Plasma Cell

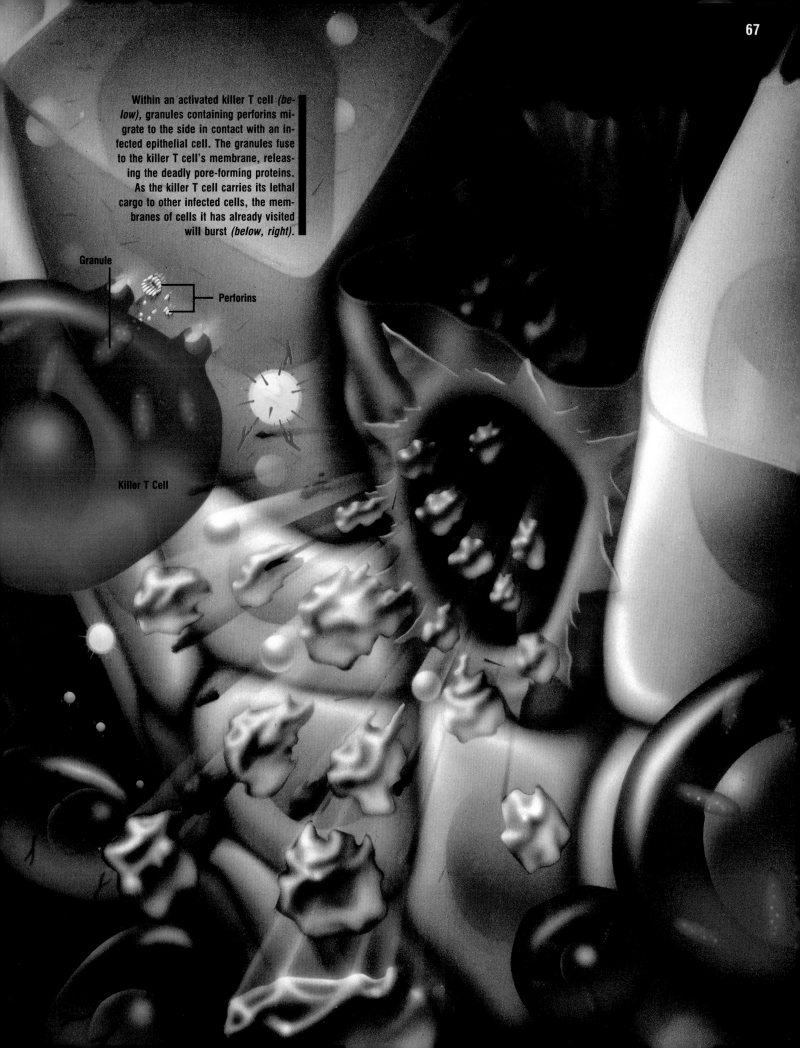

Within an activated killer T cell *(below)*, granules containing perforins migrate to the side in contact with an infected epithelial cell. The granules fuse to the killer T cell's membrane, releasing the deadly pore-forming proteins. As the killer T cell carries its lethal cargo to other infected cells, the membranes of cells it has already visited will burst *(below, right)*.

Granule

Perforins

Killer T Cell

Plasma cells *(right)* can produce antibodies for four or five days before they die. Once the viral menace disappears, no new plasma cells are created, and the output of antibodies for this specific virus begins to decline.

Plasma Cell

Memory T Cell

Memory B Cell

Memory T and memory B cells enter the blood and lymph streams as part of a recirculating pool of lymphocytes. They will patrol the body for years, ready to respond as the advance guard of a new antiviral army in the event of a second encounter with the same virus.

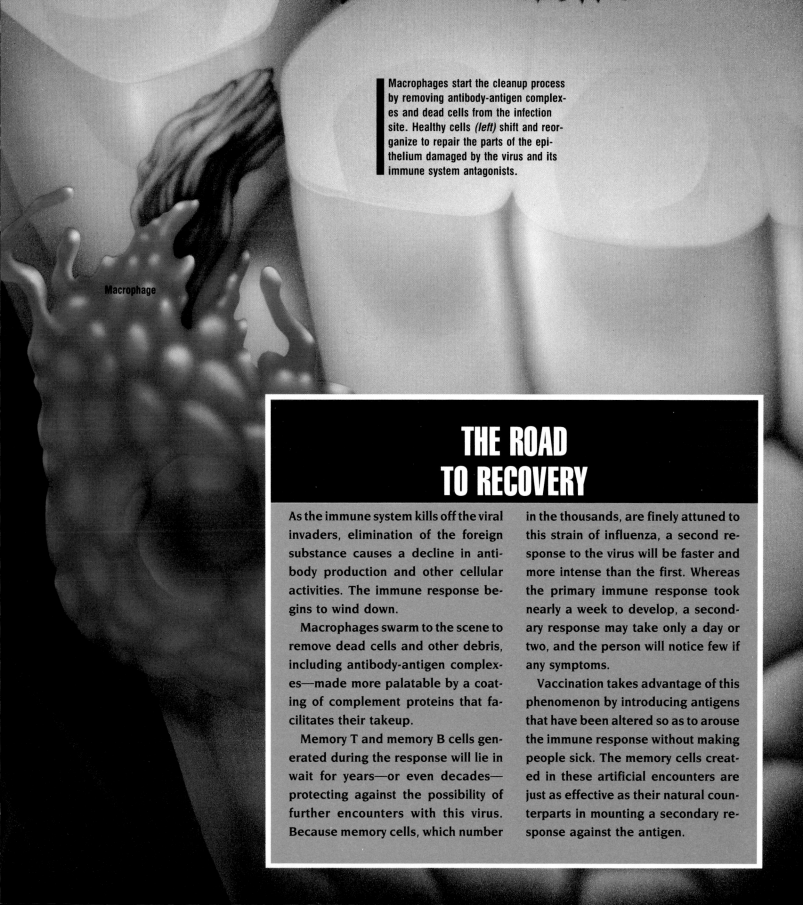

Macrophages start the cleanup process by removing antibody-antigen complexes and dead cells from the infection site. Healthy cells *(left)* shift and reorganize to repair the parts of the epithelium damaged by the virus and its immune system antagonists.

Macrophage

THE ROAD TO RECOVERY

As the immune system kills off the viral invaders, elimination of the foreign substance causes a decline in antibody production and other cellular activities. The immune response begins to wind down.

Macrophages swarm to the scene to remove dead cells and other debris, including antibody-antigen complexes—made more palatable by a coating of complement proteins that facilitates their takeup.

Memory T and memory B cells generated during the response will lie in wait for years—or even decades—protecting against the possibility of further encounters with this virus. Because memory cells, which number in the thousands, are finely attuned to this strain of influenza, a second response to the virus will be faster and more intense than the first. Whereas the primary immune response took nearly a week to develop, a secondary response may take only a day or two, and the person will notice few if any symptoms.

Vaccination takes advantage of this phenomenon by introducing antigens that have been altered so as to arouse the immune response without making people sick. The memory cells created in these artificial encounters are just as effective as their natural counterparts in mounting a secondary response against the antigen.

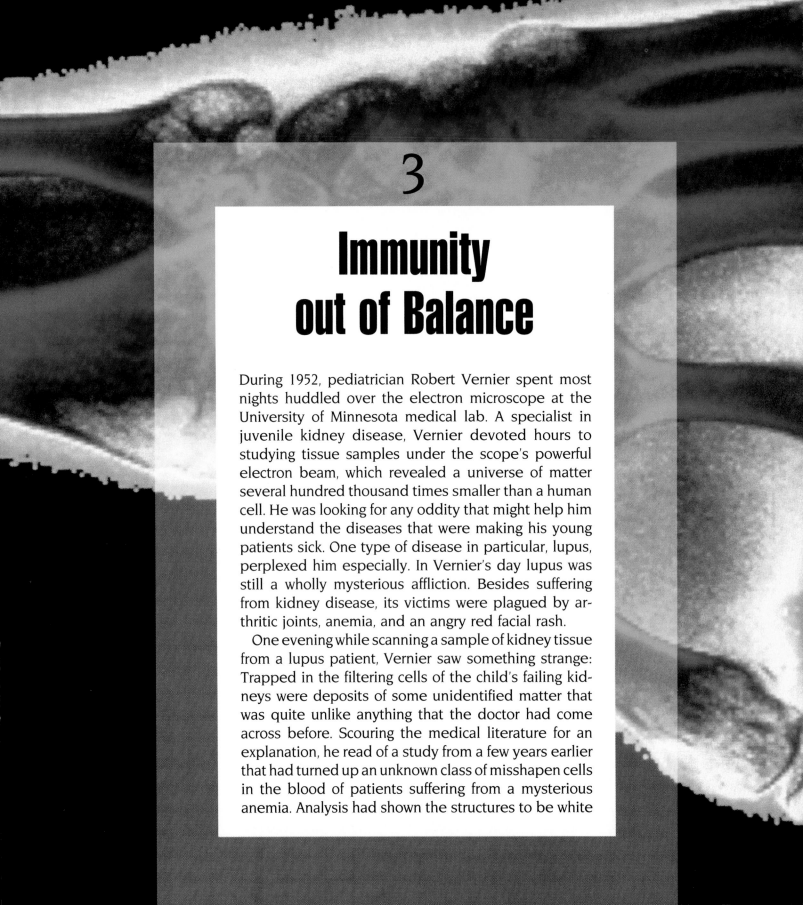

3

Immunity out of Balance

During 1952, pediatrician Robert Vernier spent most nights huddled over the electron microscope at the University of Minnesota medical lab. A specialist in juvenile kidney disease, Vernier devoted hours to studying tissue samples under the scope's powerful electron beam, which revealed a universe of matter several hundred thousand times smaller than a human cell. He was looking for any oddity that might help him understand the diseases that were making his young patients sick. One type of disease in particular, lupus, perplexed him especially. In Vernier's day lupus was still a wholly mysterious affliction. Besides suffering from kidney disease, its victims were plagued by arthritic joints, anemia, and an angry red facial rash.

One evening while scanning a sample of kidney tissue from a lupus patient, Vernier saw something strange: Trapped in the filtering cells of the child's failing kidneys were deposits of some unidentified matter that was quite unlike anything that the doctor had come across before. Scouring the medical literature for an explanation, he read of a study from a few years earlier that had turned up an unknown class of misshapen cells in the blood of patients suffering from a mysterious anemia. Analysis had shown the structures to be white

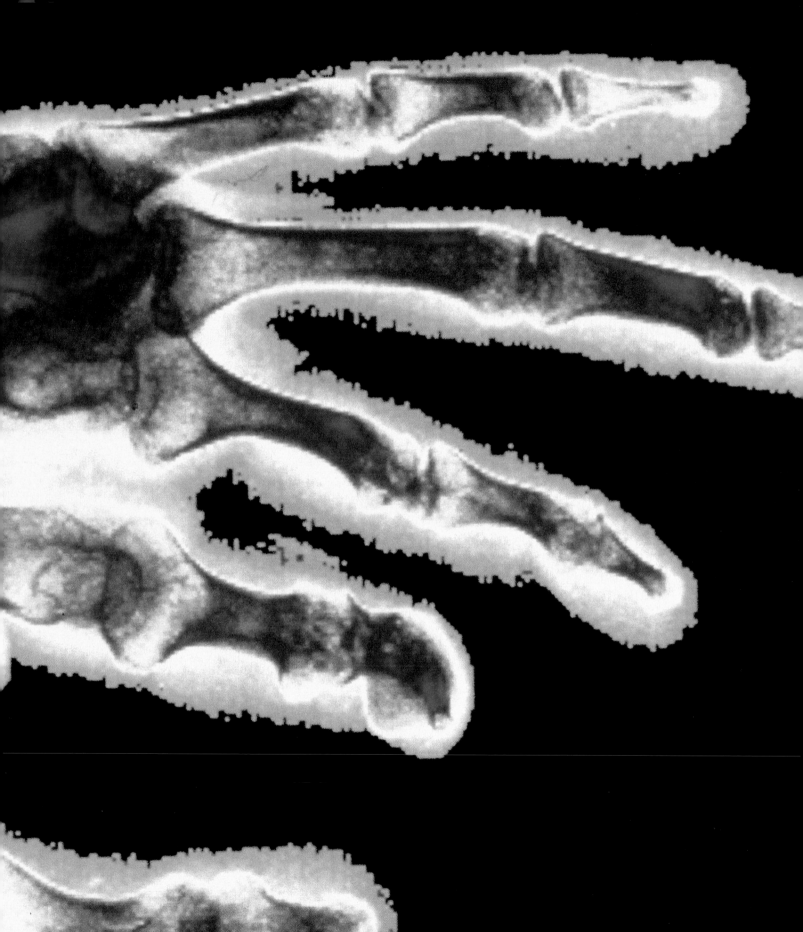

blood cells that had gorged themselves on something—exactly what remained unclear.

Vernier theorized that white blood cells might be involved in the material that was clogging his patients' kidneys. So thinking, he set about trying to discover what the cells might have ingested. First he stained the clumps from the kidneys with chemical dyes. The cells, however, resisted almost all coloration. Then a colleague introduced Vernier to a new class of fluorescent stains designed to reveal traces of rare proteins. When Vernier tried the stains on the kidney deposits, the cells turned a bright apple green, a shade that indicated the presence of immunoglobulin G (IgG), a type of antibody. Using the same dye on the abnormal lymphocytes that he had found in his patients' blood samples, he saw that these cells, too, were glutted with IgG.

Vernier was baffled. White cells do not go around gobbling up antibodies for no reason, nor do antibodies congregate in the bloodstream without cause. Yet there was no sign in these patients' bodies of an infection that might have prompted these events. What threat had the antibodies been mustered against? In time, Vernier began to think the unthinkable: Maybe the antibodies were the cause of the disease; maybe these children's immune systems had, like mutinous

troops, turned on the very bodies they were supposed to protect.

Even as late as the 1950s, thoughts such as these amounted to medical heresy. Although a few obscure afflictions had been attributed to rogue immune reactions, most physicians subscribed to the view that the human organism harbors a fundamental aversion to immunological self-destruction, an antipathy known by its Latin name as *horror autotoxicus*.

This belief was first espoused in 1901 by German bacteriologist Paul Ehrlich. He had noted that a goat injected with cells from another species developed antibodies against the foreign cells; an inoculation with the goat's own cells roused no such response. Somehow, Ehrlich reasoned, any inclination to react to the self—provided such a tendency existed in the first place—was safely quelled.

But to Vernier and a scattering of other medical researchers, matters did not seem so clear. Confronted with mounting evidence that immune cells sometimes ran amuck, these investigators continued to press their claims that failed self-tolerance, or autoimmunity, was at the root of a number of intractable diseases.

As it happened, strong evidence

that autoimmunity caused sickness was at hand. In 1948 researchers studying the blood serum of lupus patients had identified the target of the wayward antibodies. It was DNA, the building material of genes, which carry the cellular code of life. Ordinarily, the small amounts of DNA that leak into the bloodstream from dying cells during cell regeneration pose no threat. But in patients with lupus, the DNA foments an all-out immunological onslaught. Then, in the 1970s, investigators found DNA in their patients' diseased kidneys, wreathed in antibodies and engulfed by the same white cells that had attracted Vernier's attention two decades before.

Scientists have since discovered that a wide range of substances—organic or inorganic, foreign or self-made—can provoke an immune response in certain individuals. Moreover, whether that response is mounted against an infectious microbe, a drug, or an element of the person's own body, it proceeds with the same vigor. Indeed, in autoimmune diseases, deranged killer T cells and an array of autoantibodies and phagocytes destroy host tissue as if it were a lethal pathogen. Sometimes the attack is limited to a single organ, such as the insulin-producing pancreas in the case of juvenile diabetes; with other diseases, such as lupus, subversive immune cells stake

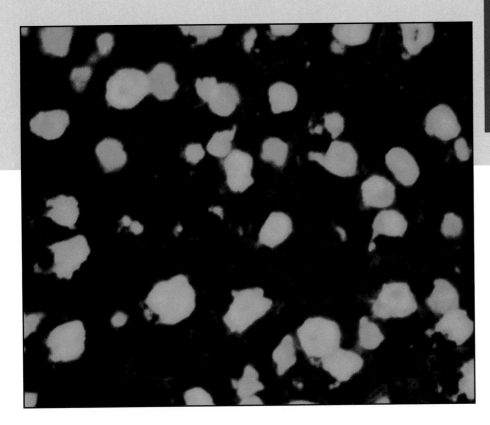

out a broad territory and ravage the body's store of DNA.

In fact, no part of the body is exempt from assault. Immunologists today recognize some 80 autoimmune disorders. Many are gravely debilitating, if not fatal, and many strike when their victims are in the prime of life. Researchers are only now beginning to unravel the complex tangle of causes and effects that characterize these bewildering disorders.

Should scientists eventually succeed in curing the many autoimmune diseases that bedevil people, they still will have won only half the battle. Each year, a growing number of individuals fall prey to another category of immune disorders: immunodefi-

ciency diseases. Unlike autoimmune diseases, which arise from an immune response that is misdirected but strong, immunodeficiency illnesses stem from crippled immune defenses that fail to protect their hosts against a variety of opportunistic infections. In one rare manifestation of this family of ailments, children are born lacking any immune system whatever, a condition known as severe combined immunodeficiency (SCID).

Much more ominous than SCID— because it is infectious and thus far more widespread—is acquired immunodeficiency syndrome (AIDS), the devastating immunodeficiency disease first recognized in 1981. In the ensuing decade, more than 2.5 million people died of the affliction; the World Health Organization estimates that many times that number now harbor the disease. Caused by the

human immunodeficiency virus, or HIV, AIDS slowly decimates the immune systems of its victims, most of whom succumb to unusual cancers and infections that most healthy immune systems would quickly dispatch. Some researchers conjecture that HIV may even invite such secondary illnesses by turning the body upon itself. In other words, AIDS may be not only an immunodeficiency disease, but an autoimmune attack on the body's own defenses as well.

Because of its rapid spread and lethal nature, HIV has become the most exhaustively analyzed pathogen in the history of the world. Researchers, though far from offering a cure, are at least zeroing in on the virus's Achilles heel—the molecular and genetic structures critical to its survival. And what they have learned has shed light not only on the dark mystery of AIDS, but also on the complex processes of immunity itself and the many ways that it affects health.

One immunological riddle investigators have solved—at least in part— centers on the questions of how and why the body manufactures autoimmune cells in the first place. Studies conducted in the early 1980s showed that, in the random process of churning out billions of T cells, the body occasionally creates a few turncoats that have the potential for attacking their host. Normally, however, these autoimmune cells—also called autoreactive cells—are killed off in the thymus, the immune system gland located over the heart where developing T cells reside until they reach maturity (*pages* 34-35). The action in the thymus is enough, in most cases, to quash any threat of insurrection. But now and then, one of the traitor cells slips free.

Everyone harbors at least a few of these rogue autoimmune cells in the blood at all times. Yet relatively few persons ever come down with autoimmune disease. Scientists believe that this is because a complex system of checks and balances normally prevents the renegade cells from doing damage. Immunologist David Hafler and his colleague Howard Weiner at Brigham and Women's Hospital in Boston speculate that in most people, some kind of suppressor cells (yet to be identified) keep the autoreactive cells in check. Whether this is, in fact, how the body polices autoimmune cells, however, is uncertain.

Far more is known about what happens when the rogue cells escape the body's controls. Hafler and Weiner spent most of the 1980s puzzling out the role of autoreactive cells in trig-

gering multiple sclerosis (MS), an autoimmune disease of the central nervous system. Victims—usually young adults—suffer symptoms ranging from slurred speech and double vision to numbness and tremors in the limbs or even paralysis. MS short-circuits the electrical signals that pass between the body's nerve cells by stripping away the protective casing, myelin, that surrounds neural fibers and enables the passage of electrochemical impulses. A type of scar tissue known as plaque grows in its place, further disrupting the transmission along the affected pathways. The type and severity of symptoms depend on what regions of the nervous system come under attack: the brain, spinal cord, or optic nerves.

Until recently, researchers had only peripheral evidence to support the theory that MS is an autoimmune disease. Although legions of T cells and phagocytes had been detected in the areas of myelin devastation in affected individuals, immunologists could not agree on whether the immune cells were the cause of—or simply a response to—the disease. In the 1930s and 1940s investigators found an animal analog for MS, a disease called experimental allergic enceph-

alomyelitis (EAE). In the years since, studies of EAE have supported the view that this disease—and, by inference, MS as well—is autoimmune in nature. Research showed that rats injected with a protein derived from myelin developed nerve damage and paralysis suggestive of MS. More important, when T cells taken from these afflicted rats were injected into healthy rats, the healthy animals came down with EAE. This experiment demonstrated for the first time that T cells could actually bring about an autoimmune disease.

In follow-up experiments, scientists isolated T cells from patients with MS and incubated the cells in the laboratory together with an extract of human myelin protein. In response to the myelin protein, the T cells began to multiply. This reaction seemed to suggest that in both EAE and MS, damage to the sheath surrounding the nerve fibers was caused by T cells that had somehow become sensitized to myelin protein.

In 1989 Hafler and Weiner identified the specific subset of T cells that they believe is responsible for the disease. However, the doctors remain unsure about what activates these myelin-sensitive cells to begin with. One popular theory holds that autoreactive T cells are drafted in response to a contagion whose surface proteins closely resemble those of a molecule made by the body—in the case of MS, myelin protein. This "molecular mimicry"—a theory first proposed in 1969 for a connection between coxsackievirus and heart disease—may fuel both an ordinary immune response against the pathogen and a misguided crossover reaction that targets the look-alike self-protein. Thus the destruction of myelin occurring in MS would be caused by autoreactive T cells, but their call to arms would first have been sounded by a virus or some other infectious agent.

There is at least one precedent in the annals of autoimmunity for such mimicry. Rheumatic fever—an inflammatory condition in which the immune system attacks the heart and joints—sometimes follows on the heels of a bacterial infection such as strep throat. As it turns out, streptococcal bacteria bear an uncanny likeness to certain molecules displayed on the cell membranes of the organs stricken in rheumatic fever.

The leading candidate for molecular mimicry in the case of MS is the measles virus. Actually, a known link between measles and MS predates the theory of molecular mimicry by nearly two decades. In the 1950s epidemiologists uncovered a quirky correlation between the geographical distribution of MS and the incidence of measles worldwide. To start with, researchers found that the farther people lived from the equator, the greater was their risk of contracting MS. Those from Minneapolis, Minnesota, for instance, were 37 times more likely to get the disease than those from Mexico City. Furthermore, children who moved from a tropical region to a temperate one before the age of 15 assumed the risk associated with their new home.

Seeking an explanation for their peculiar findings, investigators next plotted the geographical distribution of measles, a disease that most MS patients typically contracted sometime around puberty—far later than average. Intriguingly, they discovered that the late onset of measles was also linked to the world's colder regions, where MS was most prevalent.

While it was thus known that measles and MS were associated in some way, the case for a causal connection between the two was not substantially established until the 1980s, when it was found that the measles protein and myelin protein share an identical stretch of the chemical building blocks known as amino acids. Researchers conjecture that the measles virus may actually incorporate a piece of the myelin protein into itself when replicating, thus making myelin an immune system target in its own right.

Despite these provocative findings, scientists still lack conclusive proof that measles is the mimic behind MS. University of Minnesota virologist Ashley Haase has screened the brains of MS patients for the presence of measles and found that 60 percent do indeed contain the virus. On the other hand, the virus also shows up in the brains of 30 percent of people who do not have MS. More conclusive testimony that measles causes MS may have to wait until the first generation of children vaccinated for measles enters its thirties, in the latter part of the 1990s. If the incidence of MS decreases, investigators will have the confirmation they have been looking for. (However, a worldwide surge in the incidence of measles after the introduction in 1963 of a measles vaccine may confuse the issue.)

Pathogens such as measles are suspected of playing a role in several autoimmune conditions. A surprising number of self-antigens (molecules produced by the body itself that nevertheless trigger an immune reaction) have amino acid sequences similar to those found in common viral and bacterial proteins—a fact that argues

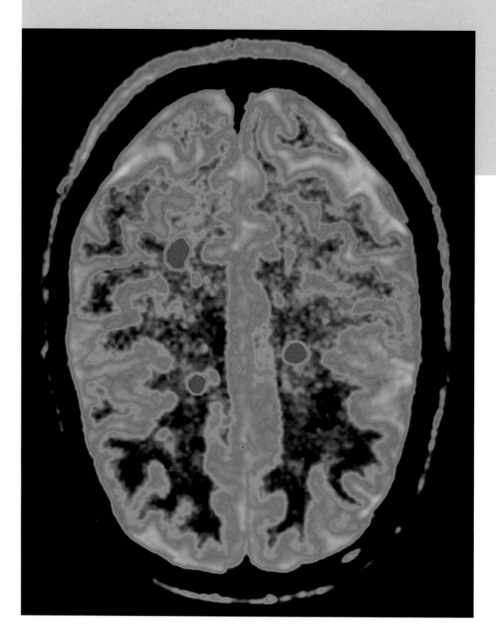

for the feasibility of the molecular-mimicry theory.

Efforts to apply the mimicry theory to lupus have produced only scant supporting evidence, however. Laboratory studies with mice and dogs suffering from a lupuslike affliction implicate a retrovirus—a type of virus that inserts its own viral genes into the host cell's DNA—in the genesis of the disease, but no such virus has been detected in the tissue of human lupus patients.

Lacking an obvious viral or bacterial trigger for lupus, many researchers have searched for leads in the runaway antibody production of its victims' B cells, the circulating lymphocytes that target antigens and destroy them by releasing antibodies. The B cells of lupus sufferers react to chemicals found in the nuclei of the body's cells, notably DNA and various nuclear proteins. As a result, the activated B cells begin spewing out antibodies that bind to this nuclear bait and form large immune complexes. These complexes eventually become lodged within the body's joints, skin, lymph nodes, spleen, liver, lungs, gastrointestinal tract, heart, and kidneys, where they foster tissue destruction and internal bleeding.

Whether an individual develops such hyperactive B cells—and hence lupus—seems to depend in large part on sex. While some victims, such as

Robert Vernier's patients, are children, most are women of childbearing age. Women, researchers find, are eight to 10 times as likely as men to contract the disease—an observation that has spurred research into the role of sex hormones in B cell activity and the development of lupus.

The earliest gender-based experiments, conducted in the 1950s, served to demonstrate the importance of hormones in promoting or preventing the disease. In one study, scientists selected mice stricken with an animal form of lupus that, like its human analog, primarily afflicts females. To thwart normal hormone production, they neutered the mice before the animals reached puberty. Researchers then gave the female

In this computer-enhanced MRI brain scan, pink areas represent damage caused by multiple sclerosis. These lesions, called plaques, result when lymphocytes and macrophages attack the myelin sheathing covering the axons, or signal-transmitting fibers, of neurons.

mice androgens (male sex hormones) and the male mice estrogens (female sex hormones). A few months into the experiment, unusually high numbers of male mice began to exhibit lupus-like symptoms of uncharacteristic severity. The females, by contrast, showed a dramatically decreased incidence of the disease, along with milder symptoms. Clearly, sex hormones have a significant effect on the progression of the disease in mice.

As subsequent research showed, they do in humans as well. Clinical studies revealed that 90 percent of all lupus victims are women at the peak of their estrogen-producing years. Moreover, males born with a congenital defect that endows them with female sex hormones are much more likely to develop lupus than normal males. Similarly, scientists say that traditionally higher levels of suppressor T cells in males may well be a critical factor in keeping autoreactive B cells in check, providing a natural deterrent to lupus.

The balance of female to male hormones appears to figure not only in lupus, but in the development of many other autoimmune diseases; overall, women are twice as likely as men to contract some of these disor-

ders, although other afflictions, such as juvenile diabetes, tend to strike men more often. But while immunologists concur that hormones figure prominently in the behavior of autoimmunity, they continue to seek a more fundamental trigger for autoimmune disease.

Philippa Marrack and John Kappler, a wife-and-husband research team at the National Jewish Center for Immunology and Respiratory Medicine in Denver, Colorado, believe they have found this basic mechanism. In 1989 the pair discovered a class of substances—toxic proteins secreted by certain deadly viruses and bacteria—that they think may be the determinant for most autoimmune afflictions. Marrack has dubbed these agents superantigens to connote their ability to impel a runaway immune response.

The path that led Marrack and Kappler to superantigens emerged in the uncharted territory of T cells, first identified during the late 1960s. As the two scientists began investigating how T cells develop and respond to different antigens in the body, much of their work focused on T cell receptors—the molecules that permit the cells to recognize invaders. Each receptor on the body's billions of T cells constitutes a kind of molecular lock, which requires a complex set of molecular keys to open.

This discovery, made by Marrack

and Kappler in about 1990, holds true for ordinary antigens. Superantigens, however, come equipped with master keys that allow them access to a broad range of T cell receptors. Whereas normal antigens activate only one in 10,000 T cells, superantigens loose one in five—or 20 percent of the body's entire detail of T cells. In one explanation of the implications of such indiscriminate arousal, Marrack likened these T cells to a kind of rogue army: "Say your body encounters one of these superantigens and Bam! it stimulates many thousands of times the T cells that would be turned on by a normal antigen. Chances are a few of those T cells are autoimmune, and now that they've been activated by the superantigen they're a lot angrier and more mobile, looking for something to attack. If they've got an attraction toward your own joints, off they go and you get arthritis."

In testing their theory, Marrack and Kappler focused on rheumatoid arthritis (RA) victims, whose wildly overstimulated immune systems suggested superantigen activity. In RA—a crippling disease characterized by chronic inflammation of the joints, heart, blood vessels, subcutaneous

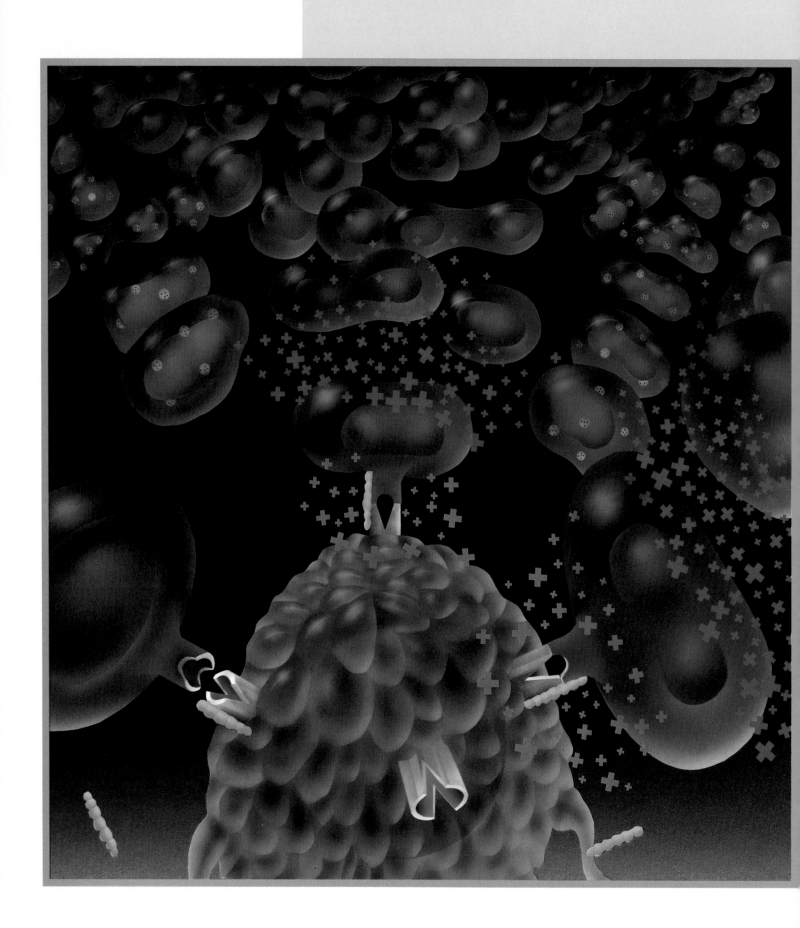

Superantigens at Work

Typically, an antigen entering the body sets in motion a chain of events that enables specific immune cells to respond appropriately to the invasion. But some foreign agents, known as superantigens, disrupt the normal processes, unleashing an overreaction by the immune system that can have dangerous consequences.

As illustrated at left, instead of being ingested by a macrophage and incorporated into its MHC-II molecule, superantigens (*green shapes*)—toxins from spoiled food, for example—bind to the outside of MHC-II molecules. Normally, only those helper T cells whose receptors matched the specific shape of the MHC-II-antigen complex would go into action (*pages 64-65*). But by attaching to the outside of receptors, superantigens activate many more T cells, regardless of the specific structure of their receptors.

Hormones (*crosses*) then stimulate a massive proliferation of more helper T cells, as well as killer T cells. The helper T cells in turn release more hormones, inducing such effects as the fever, nausea, and gastric problems associated with food poisoning. The presence of so many immune cells also greatly increases the probability of an autoimmune reaction—in which defenders attack one another or the body itself.

tissues, and lungs—the body's entire disease-fighting contingent is whipped into a frenzy of defensive action. On some unidentified cue, phagocytes, killer T cells, antibodies, and complement proteins swarm into target areas and begin releasing a barrage of tissue-destroying chemicals. Digestive enzymes discharged by white blood cells eat away at cartilage and bone, while a group of catalysts aggravates the damage by inducing inflammation.

As inflammation escalates, more immune cells rush into the fray, perpetuating the cycle of destruction. Affected areas become engorged with toxic fluids and cells that cause swelling and pain. Antibodies even turn against themselves, forming roving bands of autoantibodies called rheumatoid (R) factors. R factors lock onto other antibodies and form immune complexes that, like those in lupus, become trapped in surrounding tissues and promote further disease.

When Marrack and Kappler looked inside RA sufferers' arthritic joints, they observed an abnormal abundance of T cells that reacted to cartilage. More telling, however, was their finding that a certain subpopulation of T cells was entirely missing from the patients' blood. According to Marrack, this blank spot is the superantigen's calling card: The compounds appear not only to excite production

of T cells but also to engender the death of at least some of the very cells they excite, leaving the afflicted person's T cell count at a dangerously low level. In addition to spurring autoimmune diseases such as RA, then, superantigens may also bring on immunodeficiency.

Compelling though such findings are, the contribution of superantigens to autoimmunity has yet to be proved conclusively. Even if they turn out to be a factor in triggering RA and other autoimmune conditions, superantigens—just like the viral and hormonal agents that may be implicated in the onset of MS and lupus—cannot, by themselves, be the single cause of any autoimmune disease. Current research indicates that autoimmune afflictions result from a convergence of influences, the most fundamental of which is a genetic predisposition toward a particular disease.

Scientists have long suspected that genes play a part in autoimmunity, and statistics affirm their view: If one of two identical twins develops lupus, the other will contract the disease 50 to 60 percent of the time; the same is true of RA and of juvenile diabetes. Additionally, persons with a family history of juvenile diabetes are at 25 times greater risk of developing the disease than those from unaffected families. The link between genetics and juvenile diabetes is a particularly strong one; of all the autoimmune disorders, it has so far yielded the most striking evidence of how genes foster autoreactivity.

In juvenile diabetes, autoreactive lymphocytes descend on the pancreas, a gland located near the small intestine that functions in digestion and sugar metabolism. Painlessly, over a period of months or years, these aberrant T cells kill off the pancreatic cells that produce insulin, depriving the body of its critical supply of the hormone. Ordinarily, insulin ferries glucose from the bloodstream to the cells, which use the sugar as fuel. Without the hormone, glucose pools in the blood, where it sets off a cascade of events that can lead to premature hardening of the arteries, heart disease, blindness, and kidney failure. To escape the disease's effects, victims—most of whom suffer an onset of the disease when they are around 12 years old—must inject themselves several times daily with artificially manufactured insulin.

The genetic roots of juvenile diabetes and other diseases were first exposed in the early 1970s. At that time researchers were deciphering the immune function of the self-marker molecules—known as major histocompat-

ibility complex (MHC) proteins—that occur on the membrane of each of the body's cells. Like tiny flags, these self-markers permit the cells to distinguish self from other. MHC markers thus differ from one person to the next, though markers in individuals with similar tissue types fall into broad categories referred to as MHC types. One particular MHC type, scientists noted, showed up repeatedly in the blood of juvenile diabetics.

The researchers also noted that a person's MHC type was dictated by a select group of genes known as histocompatibility genes. These genes, they discovered, not only provide the blueprint for manufacturing the body's MHC-marker proteins, but also determine how cells of the immune system react to antigens. For instance, one form of a given gene will cause helper T cells to multiply rapidly in the face of a particular antigen, arousing a strong antibody response. In another individual, an alternate form of that same gene will boost the production of suppressor T cells, thus minimizing or extinguishing any immune response.

Although the observation that juvenile diabetics shared the same MHC type was enough to tip off scientists

that genes were a major factor in the disease, the exact role of genetics remained undefined. Pursuing a definitive link, immunogeneticist Gerald Nepom of the Virginia Mason Research Center in Seattle, Washington, in 1985 pinpointed one gene—code-named HLA-DQ—responsible for the diabetic-type MHC marker. He also zeroed in on a variation of the same gene that, in opposition to its menacing counterpart, seems to confer immunity to the disease. Later research by Dr. Hugh McDevitt and his colleagues at Stanford University unmasked three other permutations of HLA-DQ that, in some individuals, promote the disease. A fourth deviation protects against juvenile diabetes.

Immunologists now know that faulty genes predispose people to juvenile diabetes and other autoimmune diseases. Scientists surmise that the MHC self-markers in such individuals may be genetically primed to alter their own molecular structure when stimulated by certain viruses, superantigens, or environmental agents. Consequently, some part of the self suddenly appears alien, and the immune system is deceived into mounting an assault on its host body. Other genetic defects may sustain the reaction by, say, skewing the balance of suppressor and helper T cells.

Apparently, in any autoimmune disease myriad malign influences come

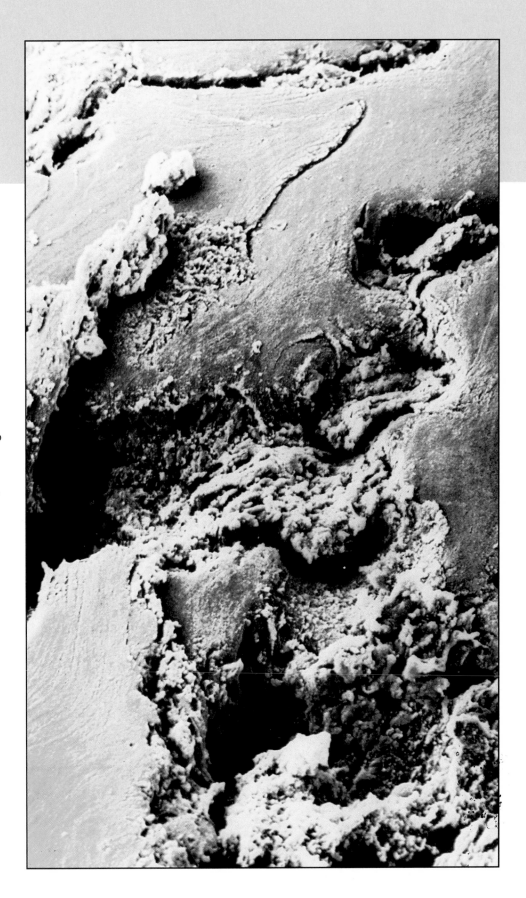

A magnified view of the surface of a human thighbone shows pitting caused by rheumatoid arthritis. Most of the protective layer of cartilage has been eaten away in a misguided assault by immune cells and associated enzymes. The resulting glut of toxic fluid in the area can produce severe swelling and pain.

into play, orchestrated by genes. The complexities involved make prospects for cures seem remote. Investigators are nevertheless putting their greater knowledge of autoimmunity to use in designing precision therapies. Like guided missiles, these treatments home in on single targets. One path of attack involves blocking chemical messengers known as cytokines, whose overproduction can precipitate an autoimmune assault. In rheumatoid arthritis, for example, scientists have fingered the chemical messenger interleukin-1 (IL-1) as a key agent in initiating inflammation. Interleukin-1, which is released by macrophages, works by docking with the receptors on lymphocytes. Biotechnology firms have engineered soluble forms of the T cell receptors for IL-1 that, in test tubes at least, prevent excess IL-1 from instigating the self-destructive response. Cytokine therapies should prove useful in treating all autoimmune disorders once the various chemical culprits at work in each disease have been identified.

Another strategy involves engineering antibodies capable of knocking out autoreactive T cells. In trials begun in the 1990s in the United States and the Netherlands, patients with RA and MS were injected with antibodies armed with toxins. As expected, the doctored antibodies went after the white cells thronging the patients' joints and nerves. Although the approach appeared to offer patients some relief, scientists caution that both diseases are prone to spontaneous remissions that might have accounted for the improvement.

Other scientists are pinning their hopes on oral vaccines. In the late 1980s a group of researchers fed rats suffering from MS-like EAE tiny bits of the myelin protein that sparks the disease. To their amazement, the rats improved markedly. Encouraged, the investigators began administering a daily portion of myelin protein to a small pilot group of human MS victims. A separate group of rheumatoid arthritis sufferers, meanwhile, began receiving dietary supplements of collagen, the protein found in joint tissue. According to its practitioners, if the therapy works, it will be much easier to use and much less expen-

sive than other high-tech treatments.

Immunologists say a true cure for autoimmune disorders will require blocking misguided immune responses at the genetic level before they can spiral into full-blown disease. Indeed, one of the most exciting developments in such therapies involves inserting new genes into autoimmune patients' DNA to reprogram their faulty immune systems. And scientists continue to learn a little more every day about what happens when the immune system turns from self-defense to self-destruction. Eventually, diseases such as lupus and MS may, like smallpox, vanish from human experience altogether.

Until the happy day when all autoimmune illnesses have been conquered, researchers are likely to find themselves increasingly wandering the borderland between immunology and genetics in search of answers. It is from that frontier, in fact, that an insight into another class of immune disorders has come.

Scientists have known for some time that the immunodeficiency ailment known as severe combined immunodeficiency (SCID) stems from a genetic defect passed from mother to

child. But they did not know the nature of the defect or how it influenced the immune system. The birth of David, who became known as the Bubble Boy, changed all that.

Only seconds after his delivery in Houston, Texas, on September 21, 1971, the chubby, dark-haired infant was whisked into a plastic isolator bubble. The death of an older brother from SCID had alerted doctors to the possibility that David might be born with the same life-threatening condition, and tests soon confirmed the worst. David, too, had the disease. Since exposure to even the most innocuous of germs could prove fatal, the decision was made to keep David inside his sterile cocoon indefinitely—at least until some attempt at a cure could be made.

Sealed away from the germ-ridden world inside a succession of hygienic enclosures, David grew into a remarkably well-adjusted child. When not at the Clinical Research Center at Texas Children's Hospital, he lived at home inside a four-room isolation unit equipped with a bed, playroom, and supply depot. The depot, which was restocked through an air lock, held an assortment of sterilized canned goods and drinks. He attended school by speakerphone, watched television, and even roughhoused with his older sister, Katherine, using the arm-length tubes attached to his bubble. Per-

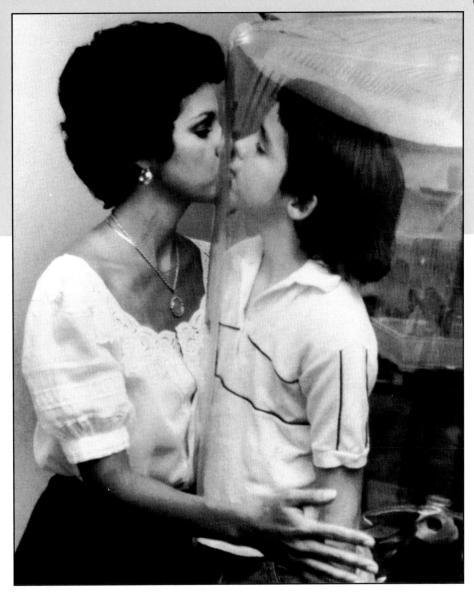

David the Bubble Boy kisses his mother through the plastic barrier that divides them. Born without any immune defenses to protect him against disease, David spent almost all of his short life in custom-designed isolation units like this one.

haps the highlight of David's short life came when he was six and NASA presented him with a battery-powered spacesuit. Thus outfitted, he ventured outside his bubble for occasional walks around the neighborhood. His ultimate dream, he said, was to run barefoot on the grass.

In 1983 new prospects for a cure seemed to bring that dream within reach. At the time, the only known remedy for SCID was a bone-marrow transplant, a procedure in which a donor's healthy red marrow—the body's source of immune cells—is infused into the patient. If all goes as planned, the donor cells take up residence in the patient's marrow, where they spawn a thriving population of lymphocytes. David had never been a candidate for the procedure, however, because no suitable donor could be found. Unless donor and recipient are the same MHC type, the transplanted cells may attack the host's tissues as foreign. The resulting graft versus host disease, or GVHD, often kills.

Sometime around David's 12th birthday, however, a new technology made bone-marrow transplants between mismatched MHC types possible. Researchers had found that the threat of GVHD could be largely

eliminated if the donor marrow was purged of mature T cells using special antibodies. David and his family decided to gamble on a better life for him and opted for the transplant.

That October, David received 1⅔ ounces of his sister's pretreated bone marrow. At first, still isolated inside his germ-free cell, he seemed to do well. But after three months or so, persistent fever, nausea, and diarrhea began to cloud his recovery. Doctors, unable to properly diagnose him inside his bubble, instructed David to crawl through an air lock into his mother's waiting arms.

The euphoria of that first touch was

quickly forgotten as, over the next 15 days, David's digestive tract ulcerated and fluid collected around his heart and lungs. On February 22, 1984, the exhausted child died of heart failure. An autopsy revealed that David had not died of graft versus host disease as expected; indeed, his sister's immune cells had never taken hold. Instead, his bowel, lungs, and spleen were clogged with clumps of abnormally large B cells of his own making. Exactly how, or why, his body mounted such an assault remains a mystery.

The tragedy of David's death has been mitigated somewhat by the legacy of knowledge that his life provided. Some 10 years after he died, cells cultured from David revealed the cause of his rare immunodeficiency disease. A painstaking analysis of David's DNA turned up a single flaw in the gene responsible for producing cell receptors for the chemical messenger interleukin-2 (IL-2). An immune system go-between, IL-2 is the lymphokine that stimulates and regulates the formation of T cells. These cells in turn secrete a growth factor that causes B cells to proliferate. Because SCID victims lack cell receptors for IL-2, the lymphokine has no receiving network to plug into, and its chemical message goes unheard. T cells never mature and B cells never get roused. The child is left defenseless.

Discovery of the genetic mutation that causes David's form of SCID offered the prospect of tests to identify women who carry the faulty gene. Even more important, this knowledge promises to spur development of gene therapies to fix the damaged gene or replace it altogether.

Genetic cures such as these are not the long shots they might seem. Indeed, gene therapy has already been put to use in treating another form of SCID known as adenosine deaminase (ADA) deficiency. Children with this disorder are born without the gene that initiates the manufacture of ADA, an enzyme that breaks down biological toxins in the bloodstream. In time, accumulated toxins kill off T and B lymphocytes, shutting down immune defenses. Such children eventually sicken and die.

In a landmark experiment in late 1990, a team of doctors at the National Cancer Institute in Bethesda, Maryland, removed a batch of T cells from Ashanthi DeSilva, a four-year-old girl afflicted with ADA deficiency. They then exposed the cells to a retrovirus whose own harmful genes had been replaced by a healthy copy of the ADA gene. As nature had programmed it to do, the retrovirus burrowed into the T cells and stitched the ADA gene into the host cell's DNA. Afterward, the T cells—each containing a copy of the newly implanted gene—were re-infused into the girl's bloodstream, where they began pumping out the missing enzyme. Within days, the girl showed an improved ability to fight disease. The following winter, when the whole family came down with the flu, she was the first to recover.

Because T cells are short-lived, DeSilva has to return periodically for follow-up treatments. Eventually, though, doctors hope to deliver the gene to the precursor stem cells that give rise to a person's lymphocytes; the child would then have a lifelong source of genetically reengineered T cells to supply her with the enzyme that she lacks.

Such miraculous therapies may ultimately be used to correct all immunodeficiencies caused by imperfect genes. But a number of other disorders, known as secondary immunodeficiencies, result from external influences that can have an equally devastating impact on the body. Malnutrition, for example, leads to immunodeficiency: In the chronically underfed, the thymus stops producing mature T cells, and the body's immune defenses begin to crumble. Certain drugs are also known to suppress immunity. Cancer patients undergoing chemotherapy, for instance, are vulnerable to a host of opportunistic infections. Even infection itself can bring on a transient immunodeficiency, as seen in individuals with common viral infections such as the flu, mononucleosis, and measles. Studies show that stress and sunlight lower immune defenses, too.

By far the most lethal of all secondary immunodeficiencies, however, is AIDS. Now a household word, this fearsome killer was not even known to exist before 1981, when the first cases were reported. Young, other-

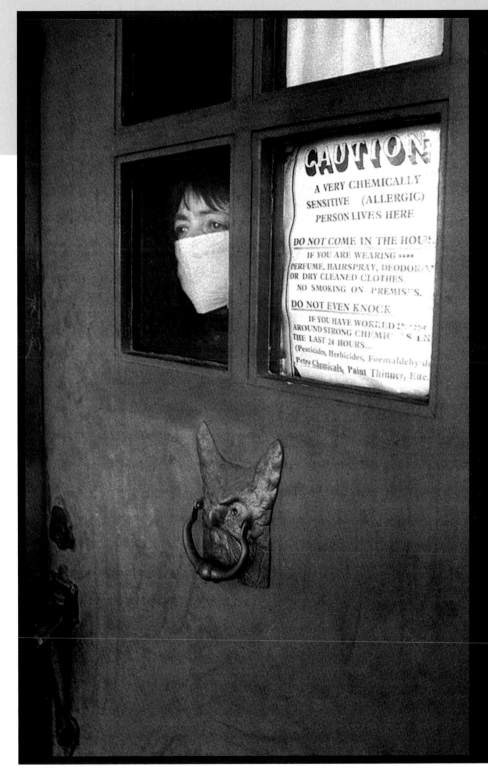

A Question of Sensitivity

Josephine Hughes (*left*) is a virtual prisoner in her own home. Only there can she effectively isolate herself from the astounding variety of common substances—from plastics to perfume—that cause her physical distress. Hughes and others diagnosed with multiple chemical sensitivities (MCS) complain of reactions including headaches, nausea, rashes, congestion, or even seizures. But the nature of the illness that afflicts them remains the subject of a controversy that divides the medical establishment.

Clinical ecologists argue that MCS stems from a single overexposure or chronic low-level exposure to chemicals that somehow throws a victim's system out of balance. Physicians, on the other hand, while acknowledging that adverse reactions to environmental substances do occur, object that there is no clear evidence of their arising from one specific ailment, stressing instead that psychological factors and perhaps a variety of unremarkable physical causes may contribute to the symptoms. To sufferers such as Hughes, however, toxins seem to be everywhere—and their bodies defenseless against them.

wise healthy men began turning up at clinics and hospitals in San Francisco, New York, and Los Angeles complaining of a bizarre constellation of symptoms: chronic fever; drastic, unexplained weight loss; swollen lymph nodes. The skin of some was mottled with reddish purple lesions. Others harbored fungal infections in the throat and respiratory tract.

Doctors diagnosed the skin ailment as Kaposi's sarcoma, an uncommon cancer that normally afflicted older men or patients taking immunosuppressive drugs. The fungal infections were found to be the prelude to a rare, deadly form of pneumonia caused by a one-celled organism. This disease, too, was seen almost exclusively in cancer or transplant patients on immunosuppressants.

By June of 1981, more than 20 men had been diagnosed with either Kaposi's sarcoma or the lethal pneumonia. Eight had died. Alarmed by the inexplicable pattern of disease, officials at the United States Centers for Disease Control in Atlanta, Georgia, convened a special task force to monitor the phenomenon. In March of 1983, the syndrome—known by then by its famous acronym—reached epidemic proportions. The number of cases was doubling every six months. Worse still, investigators had no idea what was causing it.

Early on, the only common thread epidemiologists could find linking the victims of this scourge was their gender and sexual orientation: All were gay men. Some researchers suggested that the cause of AIDS might be rooted in the victims' sexual habits; many, according to their patient histories, had been sexually promiscuous. Perhaps, the reasoning went, high-level exposure to seminal fluid—which is a known immunosuppressant—triggered the disease. Other theorists proposed that the victims' lifestyles exposed them to such a torrent of infectious agents that their immune systems just collapsed.

But such simplistic rationales were short-lived. In the fall of 1981, several heterosexual intravenous drug users were diagnosed with AIDS. Not long after that, investigators reported several cases of hemophiliacs stricken with the syndrome. Then, in what was the most revealing incidence of the disease, a San Francisco physician diagnosed AIDS in an infant who had received a blood transfusion after birth. A review of the blood-donation records disclosed that the donor was a man who had later died of AIDS.

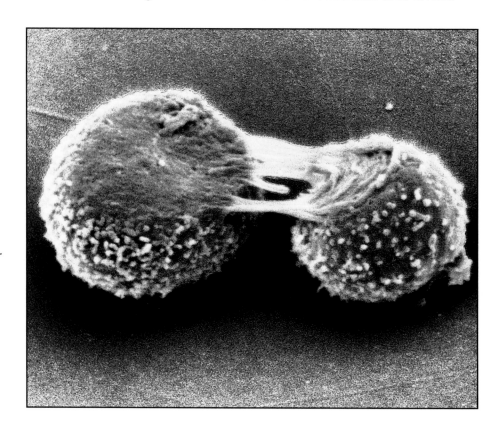

Soon there was little doubt that AIDS was transmitted by an infectious organism spread through sexual contact and blood products. To Dr. Robert Gallo, chief of the Laboratory of Tumor Cell Biology at the National Cancer Institute, the microbe's modus operandi—when viewed in conjunction with the rare cancers and opportunistic infections that plagued AIDS victims—seemed ominously familiar. Gallo had been researching retroviruses, famed for their ability to splice their own genes into the host cell's DNA. In 1980, he identified the first of two such viruses ever found in humans; the second was identified in 1982. Known as HTLV-1 and -2 (for human T-cell lymphotropic virus), the viruses foster various adult leukemias and are spread through blood and sexual contact. For Gallo, the parallels with the AIDS pathogen were too striking to be ignored. So, in May of 1982, he turned his lab's considerable resources to tracking down the mysterious microbe behind AIDS—

An experimental plasma cell, produced in the laboratory by fusing cells with different attributes, completes the act of dividing. Cells such as this have been engineered to mass-produce specific types of antibodies that, joined with radioactive markers or toxins, may be able to tag and even destroy cancer cells or errant immune cells.

one he felt sure was a close cousin to HTLV-1 and -2.

Meanwhile, at the Pasteur Institute in Paris, Dr. Luc Montagnier and a team of investigators had begun analyzing cells extracted from the swollen lymph nodes of a man in the early stages of AIDS. The scientists detected a previously unknown retrovirus in the samples. Named for the lymph glands in which it was detected, it was termed lymphadenopathy-associated virus (LAV). Montagnier's team announced its findings in an article published in the journal *Science* in May 1983, citing LAV as the probable cause of AIDS.

Gallo's investigators, who had also picked up traces of a new retrovirus in their cell cultures, made no pronouncements. Uncertain of their findings, they chose instead to wait until they had successfully isolated the virus, dubbed HTLV-3, and mass-produced it for study. Hence their findings—also published in *Science*—appeared nearly a year to the day after those of the French team. In time, LAV and HTLV-3 were found to be one and the same virus, which was later renamed HIV-1 by an international commission. Montagnier and Gallo subsequently agreed to share

credit for the organism's discovery.

Yet another AIDS virus, HIV-2, was identified by Montagnier in 1985. Not long after, investigators traced both viruses to organisms in the blood of African primates. But neither simian virus—in stark contrast to its human counterpart—makes its primate hosts sick. Somehow, perhaps in crossing the boundary from monkey to man, these viruses underwent a random mutation that rendered them deadly.

Just how deadly was demonstrated during an experiment conducted in 1984 by investigators at the National Cancer Institute. To gain insight into HIV's battle strategies, researchers first generated a batch of killer T cells that had been specially bred to destroy HIV-infected cells. At first the killer lymphocytes waged a fierce war against the diseased cells. Gradually, however, they seemed to lose their fighting edge; many stopped growing and became sluggish. When investigators examined the cells, they made a remarkable discovery: The killer T cells had themselves been infected with HIV. In time, they all died. Somehow, HIV had turned the tables. The prey had become the predator.

This strange drama, played out, in effect, in a petri dish, closely parallels the progress of HIV in the human body. Research indicates that when the body is first infected with the AIDS virus, it stages a vigorous im-

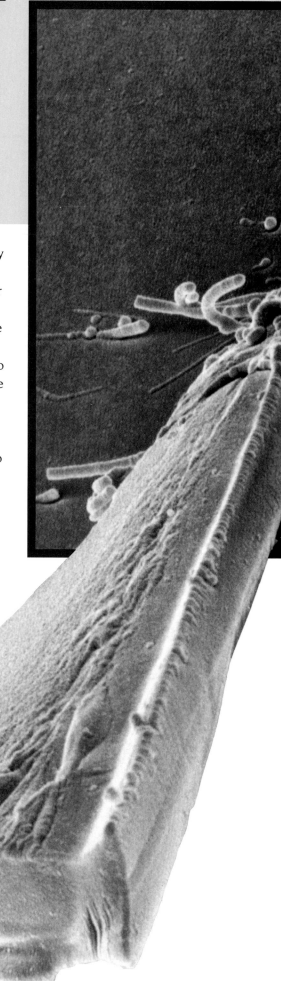

mune response, sending out wave upon wave of antibodies, killer T cells, and phagocytes. Any symptoms suffered by the victim, such as fever, fatigue, and swollen glands, quickly resolve; the immune system always wins the first battle.

It is a hollow victory, however, because the enemy has not been truly vanquished—only subdued. HIV infiltrates the body's defensive ranks, surreptitiously infecting the very immune cells that are meant to destroy it. HIV does this, many investigators believe, by slipping into macrophages and hiding itself in the cell inside small pockets called vacuoles. This is a smooth operation; no breaking and entering is involved. HIV wields a molecular key that exactly fits the receptor lock found on immune cells' outside membranes.

Once safely inside the macrophage, HIV lies dormant while its host shuttles it to the lungs, skin, spleen, bone marrow—and even the brain. Authorized to cross the semipermeable membrane known as the blood-brain barrier, macrophages are believed to act as Trojan horses that carry HIV into the cerebral cortex, the thin outer layer that is the seat of the brain's higher cognitive functions. Although the contaminated macrophages do not directly infect the brain's neurons, they apparently excrete a toxic

substance that kills off up to half of the cortical neurons. As a result, many HIV-infected persons suffer memory loss, cognitive impairment, and motor and behavioral difficulties known as AIDS dementia—often well before the actual onset of AIDS itself.

The virus-carrying macrophages also infect other immune cells, notably the body's helper T cells. A stimulus of some kind—scientists believe it may be another virus such as herpes—causes the HIV inside macrophages to abandon the vacuoles and take up residence in the cell's DNA. The virus then uses the macrophage's genetic machinery to begin producing copies of itself. Some of the new viral particles are spewed into the bloodstream, but others are passed on directly to helper T cells, when, as part of normal immune functioning, lymphocytes fuse with the diseased macrophages. Inside the lymphocyte, the virus again lies low until some-

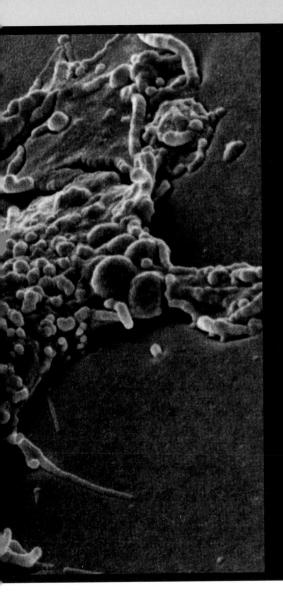

Battling against Airborne Intruders

The air we breathe is filled with all kinds of impurities, from dust, sand, and soot to asbestos fibers, minute fragments of glass and metal, and a host of dangerous chemical compounds. As the number of pollutants in the environment multiplies, the body's defenses become increasingly taxed, giving rise to reports of new types of allergies (*pages 94-99*).

When particles are breathed in, they may be repelled by first-line defenses such as the mucus and cilia that line the upper air passages and the trachea (*pages 16-19*). But irritants that are small enough can be drawn farther into the respiratory tract, even to the alveoli, the sacs of the lung where exchange of air and gases takes place. Macrophages are the main immune defenders against such intruders. The image at left shows a macrophage attempting to consume a stone flake many times its size. Such a particle would likely be coughed out, but smaller fragments that prove indigestible can become encased in tissue, forming a scar. Chronic scarring of this type characterizes many serious respiratory diseases. Moreover, the overstimulated macrophages themselves also produce a deluge of chemicals that can cause inflammation, illness, and irreparable damage to the lungs.

thing—perhaps another HIV particle—activates its host. Then HIV begins manufacturing viral clones that bud through the T cell's membrane, often bursting the lymphocyte. Unlike macrophages, helper T cells seldom survive their brush with HIV.

One of the hallmarks of HIV infection, in fact, is the decimation of the body's helper T cell population. Researchers believe HIV employs a variety of methods in killing off these defenders. The most pernicious involves the release of countless viral

keys into the bloodstream. When these keys bump up against helper T cells, they lodge in the white cells' receptors, making the cells appear infected. The hapless T cells then become the target of other immune cells—even though they are not diseased. Through such ploys, HIV not only annihilates the body's immune system elite, but also draws fire away from its own ranks.

And that is not all. HIV further confounds the immune system by altering the identifying proteins it wears on its outer coat. The virus mutates innumerable times during the course of an infection, appearing now in one guise, now in another. Some scientists

speculate that this is how HIV ultimately triumphs: When the number of virus types crosses a critical threshold, the immune system collapses, overwhelmed by the sheer diversity of viral strains in its midst.

After an average of eight to nine years, during which HIV single-handedly disarms the immune system, leaving the victims as vulnerable as infants born with SCID, the final cataclysmic phase of HIV infection begins—technically speaking, the onset of AIDS itself. The body, now virtually bereft of helper T cells, succumbs to a legion of viral, bacterial, and fungal attackers. Some 50 percent of AIDS victims who reach this stage die within a year and a half; by 18 months later, 80 percent are dead.

That is the conventional wisdom. A small cadre of scientists, however, asserts that HIV does not act alone. By itself, they say, the virus lacks the

The sequence of false-color images below shows HIV penetrating an immune cell *(1 and 2)*, then spawning new viruses that proliferate from the infected cell *(3 and 4)*. The new viruses will go on to infect surrounding cells. HIV disarms the victim's immune system by killing T cells outright and invading the DNA of other cells, where it can lie dormant for years before erupting.

resources to rout the body's entire defense force. Molecular studies reveal that, at any given time during the course of the disease, the number of HIV-infected cells in an afflicted individual is startlingly low: no more than one in 100 T cells (although other immune system cells are affected in greater numbers). Stranger still, vast amounts of circulating antibodies to HIV are found in the blood of virally infected individuals. If the antibodies are indeed combating the virus as they are programmed to do, why do these persons develop AIDS?

According to Montagnier, the codiscoverer of HIV, a primitive bacterium-like microbe known as mycoplasma may be cooperating with HIV in killing T cells, thereby enhancing immune system devastation. Another theory,

posited by Geoffrey Hoffmann of the University of British Columbia in Vancouver, holds that HIV's accomplice is the immune system itself. Hoffmann has discovered that the shape of HIV is devilishly close to the shape of the MHC molecules found on the body's own immune cells. In a stratagem borrowed from autoimmune diseases, HIV stimulates the production of antibodies not only to itself, but to the immune cells it mimics as well.

Several experiments lend provocative support to Hoffmann's supposition. One study, conducted by Hoffmann himself, showed that when a mouse was injected with ordinary immune cells from another mouse, the inoculated mouse began producing antibodies against HIV, even though neither mouse had ever been ex-

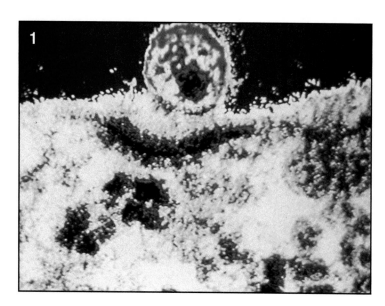

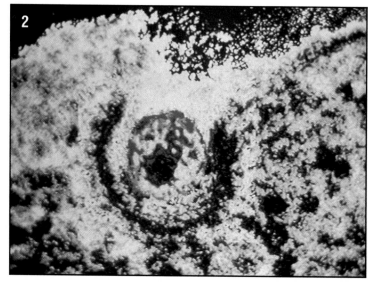

posed to the virus. This could only mean that normal immune cells bear enough resemblance to HIV to provoke an identical immune response, says Hoffmann. Similar results were obtained in an experiment with monkeys directed by E. J. Stott of the National Institute for Biological Standards and Control in Hertfordshire, England. Stott found that when macaque monkeys were injected with healthy human immune cells, they, too, developed antibodies against the AIDS virus—as did another group of macaques who actually were inoculated with live HIV.

Dani Bolognesi from the Center for AIDS Research at Duke University in North Carolina thinks he has an explanation for this phenomenon. HIV, he says, may not simply look like an MHC molecule; it may actually be stealing MHC molecules from the cells it infects and using them like molecular camouflage. The body's immune response, then, is directed against these pilfered MHC proteins rather than against the virus itself. That is why inoculation with normal immune cells induces the same immune response as infection with HIV.

The curious findings of Hoffmann and Stott suggest that HIV is only the spark that touches off the self-immolation recognized as AIDS. In this scenario, AIDS is not an immunodeficiency disease but an autoimmune disease afflicting the immune system itself.

To Bolognesi, these findings also suggest a novel possibility for creating a vaccine against AIDS. People could be protected against AIDS, Bolognesi says, by the injection of a cocktail of MHC proteins. If the experiments with mice and monkeys are any indication, this should generate antibodies to the MHC molecules that would also attack HIV.

To the majority of scientists, however, this sounds far-fetched, if not downright dangerous. While many find the autoimmune model for AIDS intriguing, most back the more orthodox vaccines and therapies built around traditional models of AIDS. The most widely used AIDS therapy has been azidothymidine (AZT), a drug that interferes with HIV's ability to replicate itself. After about 18 months, however, AZT's efficacy drops off because the virus mutates into a form that is less susceptible to the

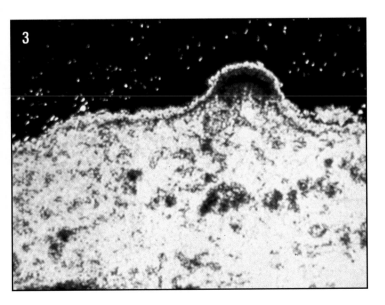

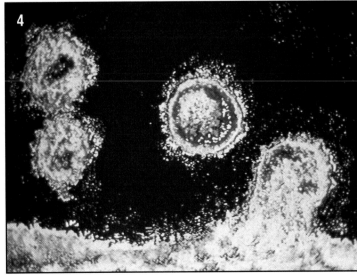

drug. Moreover, the drug is also extremely toxic to bone marrow, severely inhibiting the production of both red and white blood cells. Not surprisingly, dozens of pharmaceutical companies around the world are locked in a race to develop more effective treatments and vaccines.

Developing preventive vaccines has been even trickier. The fear that using the traditional medium of vaccination—killed or inactivated HIV particles—could somehow trigger AIDS has driven most researchers to create vaccines that use only fragments of the virus to stimulate an antibody response. (Some preliminary research has been done, however, with both live and killed vaccines.) One vaccine design developed at the University of California at San Diego uses a piece of HIV's protein coat to foster immunity; another uses the gutted shell.

Other therapeutic vaccines are being designed to kick-start the immune systems of those already infected with HIV. Jonas Salk, the developer of the first polio vaccine, has created a therapeutic AIDS vaccine made up of HIV's core proteins. Salk believes the vaccine will strengthen the body's T cell response, helping to delay or prevent the onset of full-blown AIDS.

Scientists are guardedly optimistic about the prospects for ultimately managing AIDS. Effective treatment, they say, will doubtless lie in a combination of therapies rather than in any one wonder drug or vaccine. Hopes for a total eradication of the scourge are probably unrealistic, however; no sexually transmitted disease has ever been entirely extinguished.

And clearly, despite a mammoth research effort across the globe—involving an unprecedented marshaling of modern science's resources—there is still much that scientists do not understand about this terrible affliction. One of the deepest mysteries confronting investigators is why a tiny percentage of HIV-infected persons fail to come down with AIDS—even when, as their patient histories reveal, more than 14 years have elapsed since their initial exposure to the virus. Scientists have documented at least 70 such cases.

Researchers theorize that there may be something different about the way the immune systems of these individuals respond to the disease; or that their bodies are grappling with a weaker strain of the virus. But in many of these patients, there seems to be another factor at work: a positive mental attitude. Michael Leonard, a floral designer from Los Angeles, was diagnosed with AIDS-related complex in 1985. Eight years later he was still getting up at 5:00 a.m. each day, meditating, and putting in a full day at work. After work, he would head for the bowling alley or an evening at the movies with friends.

When asked why he was doing so well, Leonard responded, "It's not because of medicines, because I haven't taken pharmaceutical drugs for seven years. It's not because of doctors, because I haven't empowered them to run my life.... I think it's because I haven't time to die. It takes too much work to die."

Ron Webeck of St. Petersburg, Florida, also diagnosed in 1985, appears to be another whose positive attitude has kept him going longer than any-

one would have expected. "I just decided one day that I'm not going to die," he once said. To heal himself, Webeck—at the time gravely ill with a secondary viral infection—set himself a series of simple goals like getting out of bed, walking across the room, and going around the block. He recovered. According to Webeck, "What keeps me alive is the feeling that I can't let other people down. The more people I help, the better I get."

Testimonies such as these have prompted medical professionals to explore more fully the mind's relationship to immunity. What they have learned is revolutionizing the way these caregivers define illness, as well as how they go about sustaining health and combating disease.

"It's not because of medicines.... It's not because of doctors.... I think it's because I haven't time to die. It takes too much work to die."

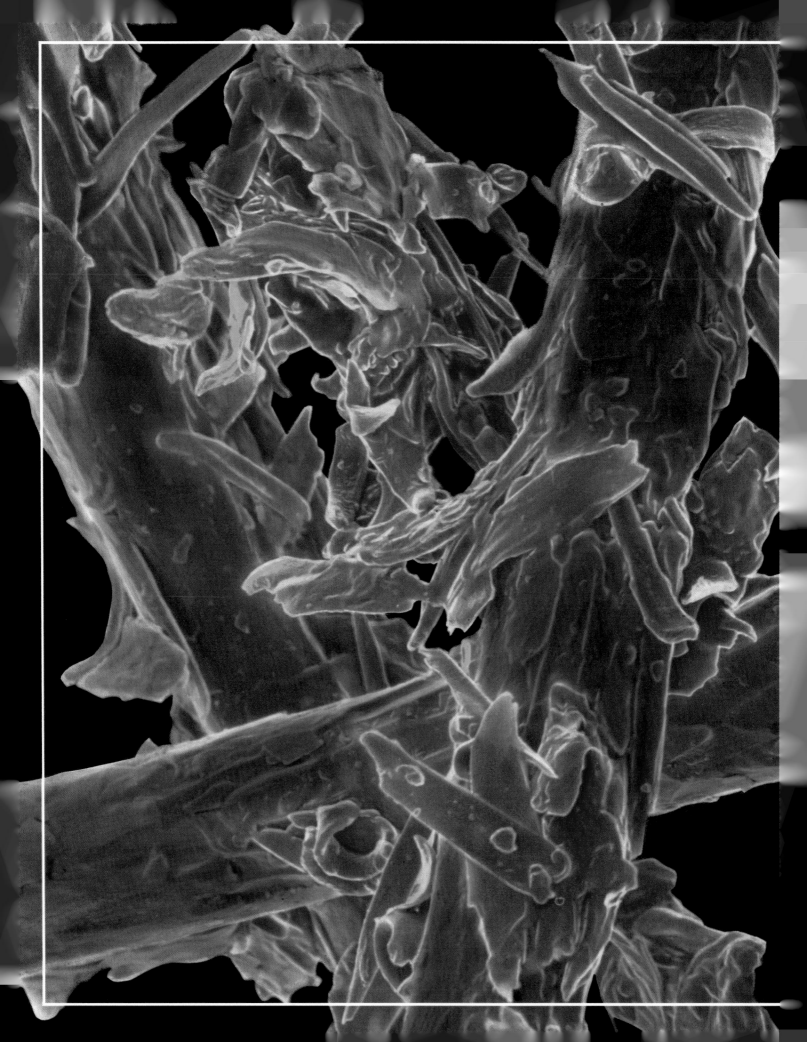

A TRIO OF ALLERGENS. Three electron micrographs offer closeup views of some allergy-causing substances, or allergens, each magnified more than 700 times: flakes of dander among dog hairs *(left)*; penicillin *(below)*; and grains of dandelion pollen *(bottom)*.

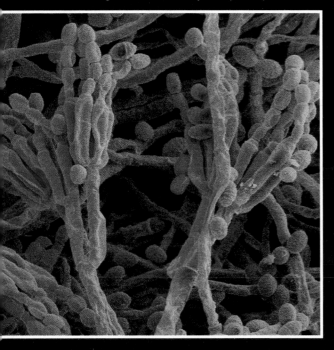

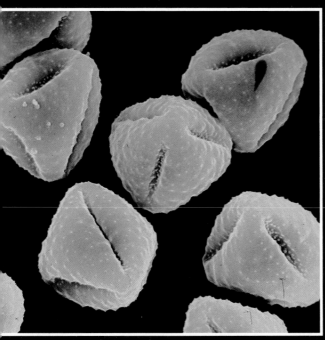

SENSITIVE TO A FAULT

In its zeal to protect the body from pathogens, the immune system often mistakes harmless substances for dangerous ones and reacts accordingly. Perhaps the most familiar over-reaction, or hypersensitivity, is the allergy. In many people, for example, pollen grains, animal dander, and other essentially innocuous substances trigger an immune response that results in the itchy, watery eyes and sneezing fits of hay fever.

Although hay fever is rarely life-threatening, other allergic reactions can be. Those allergic to bee venom, for instance, can die from a sting in minutes. Severe reactions are also possible in people allergic to certain drugs and foods.

Not surprisingly, allergies appear to be strongly influenced by genetics. The tendency to be allergic—though not necessarily to particular substances—may be passed from one generation to the next. In recent years scientists have also found a mental, or psychological, component to these reactions. Hypnotized subjects, for example, may show a physical reaction to ordinary ivy if told that it is poison ivy, and people who suffer allergic asthma may have more severe attacks if they are under stress.

THE STORY OF AN ALLERGIC REACTION

Allergens may be inhaled or eaten, or they may penetrate through the skin. The foreign substance may be quickly digested by a macrophage or B cell, which can misidentify the allergen as a dangerous pathogen, thus setting off the chain of events described in

simplified form below. The result is the production of the antibodies immunoglobulin M (IgM) and immunoglobulin E (IgE), both created to fit the particular allergen.

The manufacture of IgM soon stops, but these antibodies will now bind to

any free-floating allergens, thereby flagging them for destruction by macrophages. The IgE antibodies, for their part, bind to basophils in the bloodstream and to mast cells in nearby tissues. Thus sensitized, basophils and mast cells are now primed to

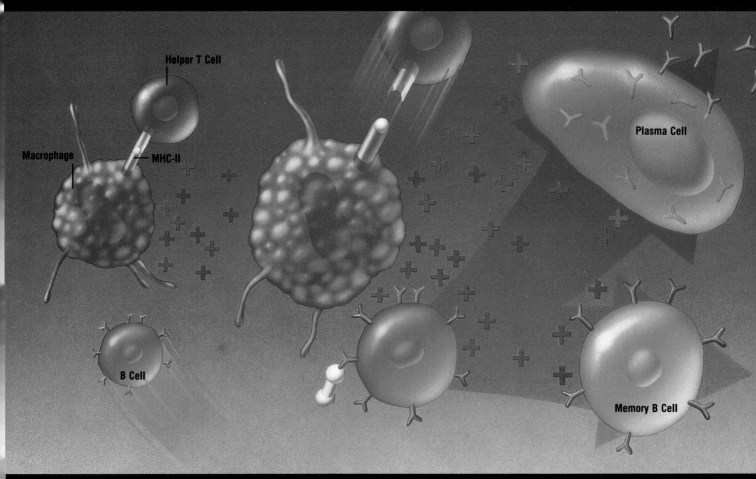

SENSITIZATION. When an allergen first enters the body, it may be consumed by macrophages *(blue)*. Proteins from the digested allergen *(yellow ball)* bind to MHC-II receptors and migrate to the macrophage surface, triggering the release of cytokines *(blue crosses)* that attract helper T cells *(purple)*. These briefly bind to the MHC-II-allergen complex and then

release their own cytokines *(purple crosses)*.

When nearby B cells *(green)* encounter an unprocessed allergen *(yellow barbell)*, the allergen binds to any antibodies *(green Ys)* on the B cell that fit the allergen's molecular configuration. With the help of cytokines released by helper T cells and the macrophage, the B cells begin to multiply. As the growing army of

B cells mature into plasma cells *(green oval)* and memory B cells *(light green)*, plasma cells begin churning out IgE antibodies. The IgE, which fits the specific allergen, then binds to a mast cell *(orange)*, sensitizing it for future encounters with the invader. Plasma cells are active for three to five days; memory B cells remain at the ready for as long as 40 years.

react to any future encounter with this allergen. The next time, these sensitized cells will release chemicals called mediators of inflammation, causing blood vessels to dilate and enabling immune cells to rush to the attack of the allergen. The attack is what produces the physical symptoms of allergies.

In the case of common pet and pollen allergies, small quantities of mediator chemicals released in the tissues of the respiratory tract result only in sneezing and watery eyes—hay fever. But with bee-sting and some food and drug allergies, large quantities of mediators are released into the bloodstream, allowing them to travel throughout the circulatory system. This produces systemic anaphylaxis, a fast-acting and often fatal reaction.

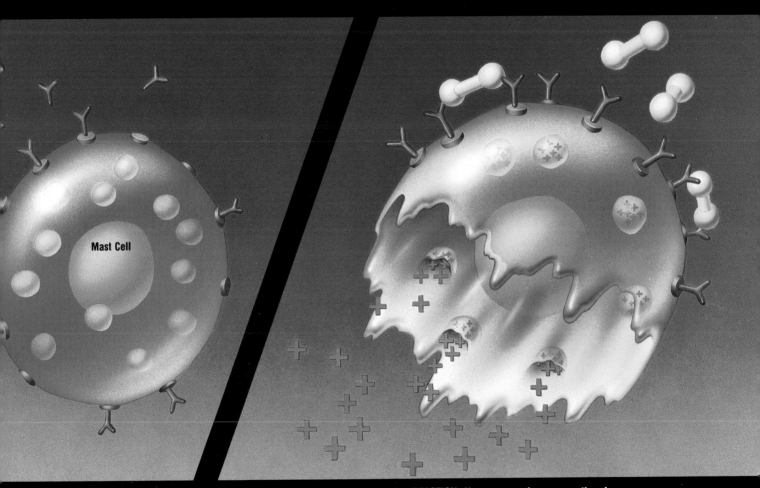

Mast Cell

REACTION. Upon a second exposure, the allergen will meet a sensitized mast cell. As it binds to and links at least two IgE antibodies on the cell's surface, the allergen completes an electrochemical circuit that causes the cell to rupture, releasing the chemical mediators *(orange crosses)* that generate the physical symptoms of a reaction.

HEADING ALLERGIES OFF

Although shunning the offending substance is the best way to prevent allergic reactions, not all allergens are easily avoided. To reduce the severity of reactions when they do occur, many people undergo a series of allergy-shot treatments. After determining through trial and error what allergen the patient reacts to, the doctor injects a pure dose of the specific protein in the allergen that causes reactions. The shots are repeated twice a week and then at less-frequent intervals, usually for up to a few years.

Allergy shots are believed to work for two reasons. First, an injection of pure allergen stimulates production of immunoglobulin M (IgM) and immunoglobulin G (IgG), rather than IgM and IgE. As shown below, IgG works to block the immune response the aller-

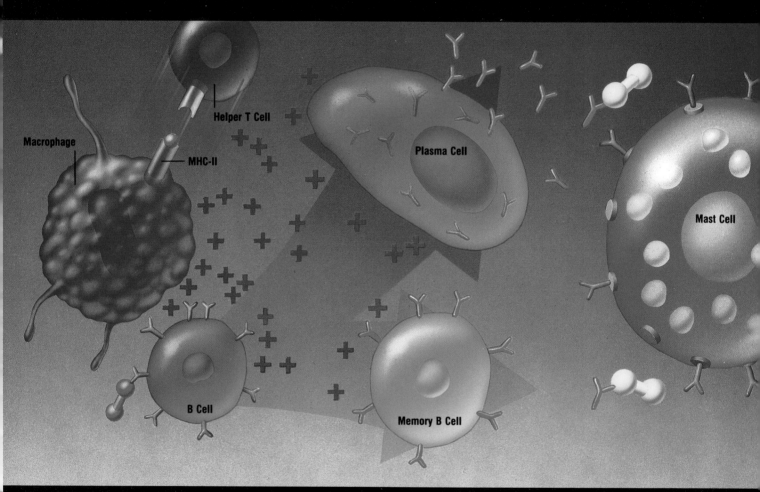

AN ALLERGY SHOT. Injection with a pure allergen *(red barbell)* causes an immune response virtually identical to that of an allergic reaction, except that newly created plasma cells *(green oval)* produce the antibody IgG *(red Ys)* instead of IgE.

PREVENTING A REACTION. The next time the allergens appear, IgG antibodies bind to them before the allergens can attach to the IgE antibodies on sensitized mast cells. The efficiency of this process varies from person to person, which is why allergy shots are not equally effective for everyone.

gen would normally generate. Second, repeated doses somehow desensitize the body to what would be regarded as nonself, thus making an immune response unnecessary.

Allergy shots are not always the answer, however. Only five percent of those receiving shots are fully desensitized to allergens, and for many the shots are entirely ineffective. A treatment that holds greater promise is one with "anti-IgE antibodies," proteins that bind to IgE, preventing it from binding with the allergen.

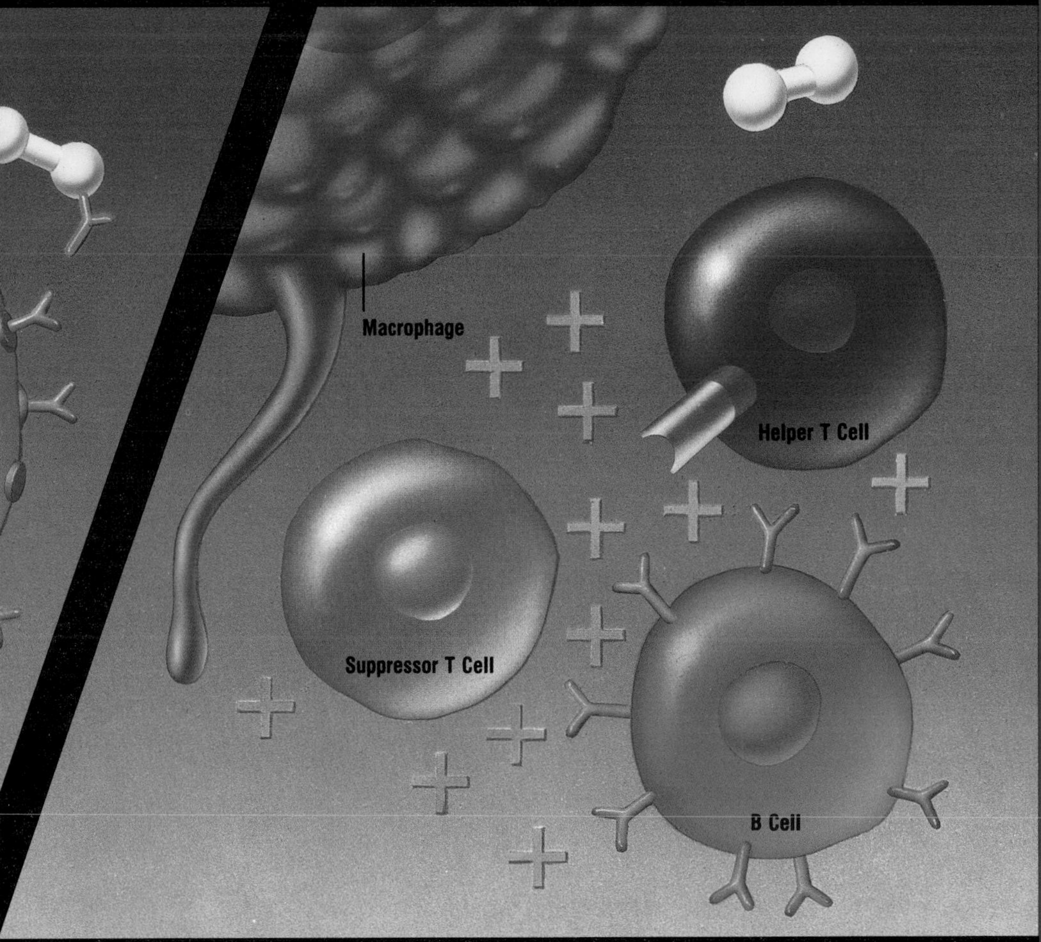

PROLONGED RESISTANCE. After years of allergy shots, the body may come to accept the presence of the allergen. Scientists theorize that, as a result, suppressor T cells *(light purple)* release cytokines *(light purple crosses)* that prevent B cell proliferation and also keep helper T cells from initiating reactions every time the allergen appears.

FOUR TYPES OF ALLERGIC REACTIONS

Hypersensitivities generally fall into one of four types, labeled I through IV. Although physicians treat each type as a distinct affliction, a given reaction often contains elements from more than one type.

Type I hypersensitivities are common allergic reactions, in which immunoglobulin E is produced. Types II and III on the other hand, which are commonly triggered by drugs such as penicillin and by dairy products, begin when foreign invaders, or antigens, bind to cells within the body's tissues and organs. Antibodies then attach to the antigens, marking them for attack by macrophages.

In the course of their assault, the macrophages also destroy the cells to which the antigens are attached. Minimal tissue destruction occurs in type II reactions, but type III reactions can wreak widespread damage. Both types of reactions may also lead to so-called autoimmune disorders, such as certain types of anemia in the case of type II and rheumatoid arthritis in type III.

Type IV reactions, also known as contact hypersensitivities, arise when a substance comes into direct contact with the skin. Common offenders in this case are poison ivy and poison oak, as well as certain industrial chemicals and metals.

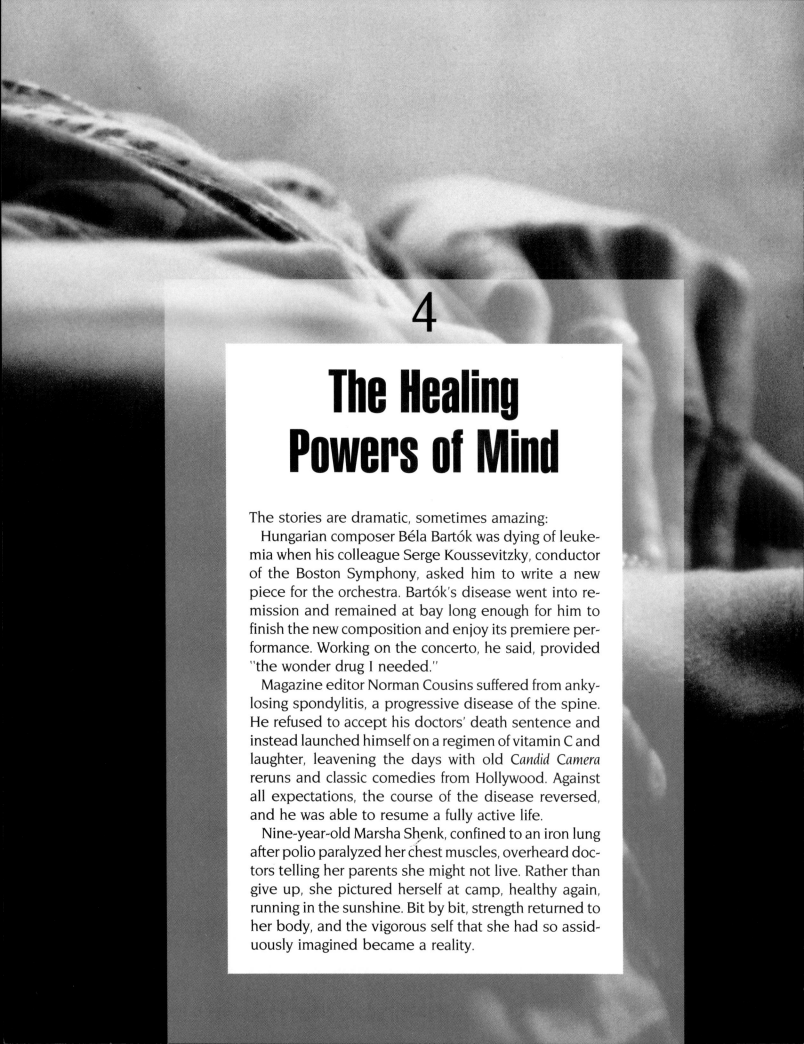

4

The Healing Powers of Mind

The stories are dramatic, sometimes amazing:

Hungarian composer Béla Bartók was dying of leukemia when his colleague Serge Koussevitzky, conductor of the Boston Symphony, asked him to write a new piece for the orchestra. Bartók's disease went into remission and remained at bay long enough for him to finish the new composition and enjoy its premiere performance. Working on the concerto, he said, provided "the wonder drug I needed."

Magazine editor Norman Cousins suffered from ankylosing spondylitis, a progressive disease of the spine. He refused to accept his doctors' death sentence and instead launched himself on a regimen of vitamin C and laughter, leavening the days with old *Candid Camera* reruns and classic comedies from Hollywood. Against all expectations, the course of the disease reversed, and he was able to resume a fully active life.

Nine-year-old Marsha Shenk, confined to an iron lung after polio paralyzed her chest muscles, overheard doctors telling her parents she might not live. Rather than give up, she pictured herself at camp, healthy again, running in the sunshine. Bit by bit, strength returned to her body, and the vigorous self that she had so assiduously imagined became a reality.

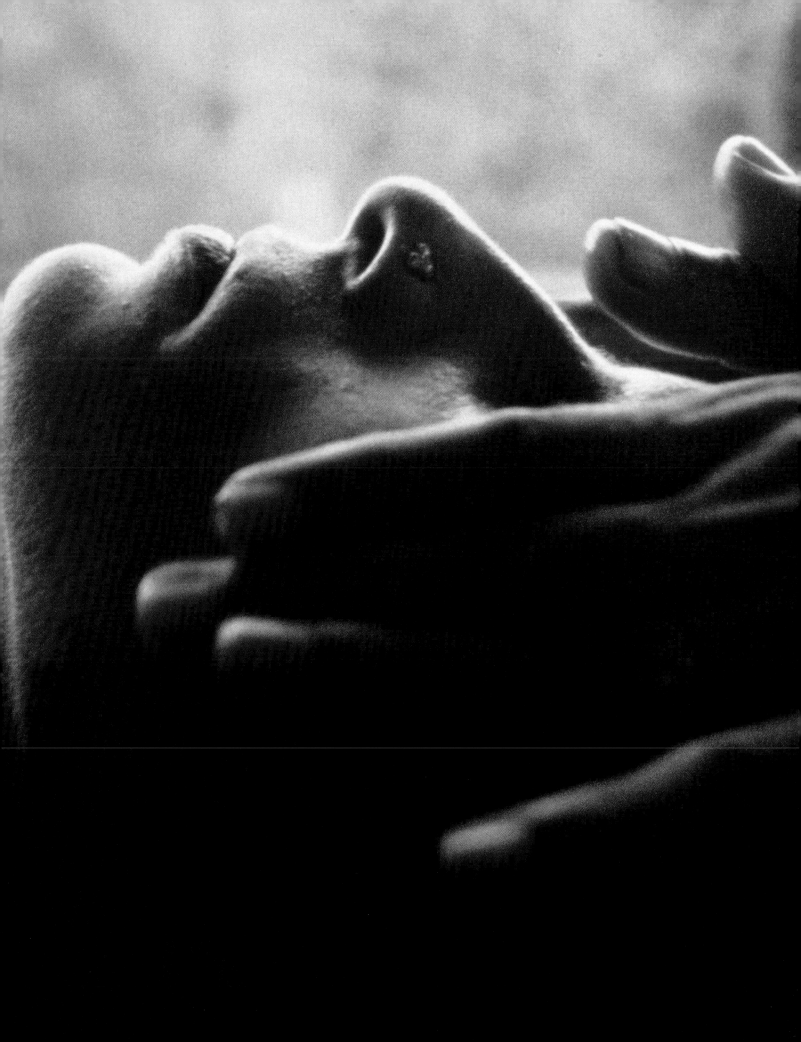

Such cases (and there are thousands) seem to indicate that the thoughts and emotions of a sick person can play a major, perhaps decisive, role in the body's response to the illness. In the entire wonder-filled world of modern medicine, no idea is more exciting. The evidence that healing is a joint endeavor of body and mind could lead to new treatments and a fundamentally altered relationship between patient and doctor. On the other hand, it may be that hopes of enlisting the mind as an active partner in all types of healing are more wishfulness than attainable reality. Sorting out the facts and pursuing the implications of this mind-body matter ranks as one of the top priorities in medical research today.

Since ancient times, physicians have suspected that people's state of mind is somehow related to their susceptibility to disease. In the second century AD, for example, the Greek physician Galen noted that "melancholic" women—those who nowadays would be called passive, or depressed—seem more likely to develop breast cancer. Now medical investigators are turning such enlightened guesses into statistics. Recently, for instance, a British study of breast-cancer patients appeared to buttress Galen's observation (although only approximately, because it dealt with recovery rates

rather than incidence of cancer). The study, based on 10 years' worth of results, found that the women who remained cancer free after treatment tended to be those who met the disease with a fighting spirit; by contrast, those who accepted their diagnosis with stoicism, resignation, and helplessness were more likely to suffer a recurrence or to die during their first bout with the cancer.

Doctors have also long known that a patient's expectations can influence the healing process. One of the clearest medical links between body and mind is the phenomenon known as the placebo response. A placebo (Latin for "I shall be pleasing") is a medically inert substance—a sugar pill, for instance—that is presented to a patient as possessing therapeutic value. Until only a few decades ago, placebos, slyly labeled Obecalp (placebo spelled backward), were part of the pharmacopoeia of many family doctors. Blue sugar pills were given to soothe the nervous, orange ones to invigorate the run-down, and they often seemed to help. Today, more-effective medications are available, and in any event, the law requires drug manufacturers to prove the medical merit of their products. Nonethe-

less, research into the phenomenon continues—and with good reason. One study determined that, for almost any disease, a third of the symptoms abate when a patient receives a pharmacologically inert placebo treatment. A related finding is that placebos help 35 percent of patients receiving them. Some recent research suggests that the percentage of patients benefiting from placebos will double when the treatment is given in an enthusiastic way by a trusted physician.

Belief in the efficacy of the treatment is the key to the placebo response, and it need not center on a substance. Each year, more than four million pilgrims journey to the Shrine of Bernadette in Lourdes, France, hoping to be cured of their ills through spiritual intervention. Although the Vatican has certified fewer than 100 miraculous cures at Lourdes, more than 6,000 believers have proclaimed themselves healed by their visit to the shrine. Some medical researchers see Lourdes as an institutionalized version of the placebo response. Similarly, they speculate that shamans, faith healers, and numerous other practitioners outside the mainstream of Western medicine achieve some genuine successes because of their patients' belief in the possibility of a cure and the authority of the curer.

Several decades ago, a case involving a drug called Krebiozen suggested that the placebo response can turn on and off almost like a light switch. Although Krebiozen has since been discarded as medically worthless, it stirred high hopes when it was being tested as a cancer treatment in the United States during the 1950s. One man, terminally ill with advanced lymphosarcoma, asked to be given Krebiozen after he heard that it was a promising anticancer weapon. His

doctor obliged and reported that the patient's tumors "melted like snowballs." The patient returned to work and resumed his normal life. Some months later, however, he read news reports calling the substance worthless. His health collapsed again, and death loomed. But his doctor, feeling the man's failing condition justified a deception, told him that a special, pure form of Krebiozen was effective and had become available. He inject-

Doctors made up as clowns cheer Jackie Vittini (in the oversize spectacles and bushy eyebrows), recovering from third-degree burns over most of her body. Not only may a good laugh alleviate the stress of hospitalization, but a positive mood in general is thought to help the immune system work more efficiently.

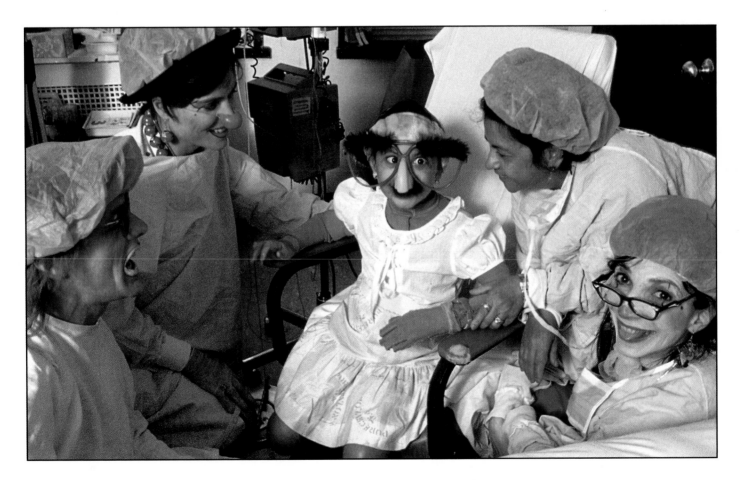

ed the patient with distilled water. Once again, the patient made a remarkable recovery. Then, two months later, the man read a government report declaring that Krebiozen, in any form, was absolutely worthless. Stripped of his belief once more, he suffered an abrupt relapse and died within days.

The placebo effect represents just one sector of medicine's mind-body frontier. As on all frontiers, the picture of progress is confusing, with many contending claims and numerous heated disputes. Some of the pioneers have concentrated on devising new approaches to treatment rather than on systematic investigation of the terrain. In the late 1960s, for example, American oncologist Carl Simonton, discouraged with the standard cancer-fighting tools of radiation and chemotherapy, began pondering the healing powers of the mind as he observed dozens of patients recover their health in spite of dire medical predictions. The secret of these people who refused to die, he felt, was imagination, a positive outlook, and will power. He and his then-wife, psychologist Stephanie Simonton, set up the Cancer Counseling and Research Center in Dallas, one of many so-called holistic health centers then opening across the United States. (The term *holistic* refers to a philosophy of treating the patient as a whole

person, rather than simply focusing on the disease process.) Through counseling and other methods designed to increase self-awareness, the Simontons trained cancer patients to confront their social and emotional problems, to face their illness with determination and hope, and to use mental imagery against the disease—visualizing cancer cells being demolished by fierce attack dogs or unerring bullets, for example. In a book published in 1978, they reported some impressive results with a total of 159 patients. At the time of diagnosis, they said, all of the patients had been given less than a year to live, yet most survived for at least 20 months. Some recovered completely.

These claims were generally ignored or dismissed by the medical establishment. Skeptics questioned whether all of the supposedly "terminal" cases had been diagnosed correctly; they pointed out that some patients had been well enough to travel to the clinic from great distances. Doubters also noted that the clinic's program of teaching patients to "take control" of their lives may simply have increased the chances that they would follow doctors' orders properly. There was an ethical issue,

as well: The assertion that survival depended upon mental strength seemed to imply that failure to recover was somehow the patient's fault.

In considering claims by the various apostles of mental healing—clinicians like the Simontons, authors like Norman Cousins, enthusiasts in the media—the chief concern of the medical mainstream was that high hopes were being constructed on a very uncertain scientific foundation. Such evidence as recovery rates in holistic treatment centers or personal accounts of healing by laughter could be highly misleading, many physicians feared. Considering the well-documented existence of the placebo effect, no one could deny that the mind has the capacity to induce physiological responses in the body. But how does such a thing occur? And when? And what are the limits? Most medical researchers advised caution until solid facts replaced the many unknowns—not least, the unknown mechanisms that might enable the brain to control the body's disease-fighting weapons. As one physiologist at the National Institutes of Health (NIH) in Bethesda, Maryland, put it: "In science, credibility depends on opening up the black box and finding out what's inside."

Logic strongly suggested that the hidden mechanisms involved the immune system. But until just a few dec-

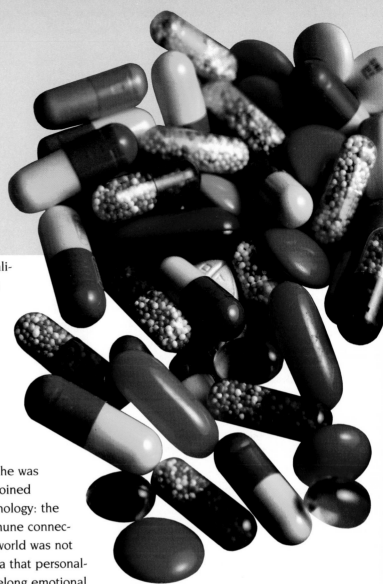

Bright hues can actually enhance a pill's prescribed effects—a phenomenon called the placebo response. Blues and greens, for example, have a calming influence; oranges, yellows, and reds are stimulating. Shape, texture, and taste have also been found to contribute to the impact of vitamins or medicine.

ades ago, medical orthodoxy held that this was unlikely. As a deeper understanding of the immune system gradually emerged in the 1960s, researchers tended to view it as splendidly autonomous. Marveling at the intricacy and flexibility of the defenses, most decided that, alone among the body's systems, the immune system operates on its own, unaffected by the brain. But there were some doubts early on. In 1964 psychiatrist George Solomon and his associates at Stanford University announced that they had identified specific emotional influences in the development of rheumatoid arthritis, an autoimmune disease. Their subjects were a group of women all genetically predisposed to develop the painful, joint-eroding affliction, which occurs when the immune system attacks cartilage as if fighting an infection. Some of the women, however, were disease free, and the research team attributed their health to nonphysical reasons: "They were not depressed," Solomon said; "they were not alienated. They had good marriages. We felt that emotional health protected them from rheumatoid arthritis."

Solomon was building on earlier work that suggested the existence of a "rheumatoid personality," one that represses anger and expresses other emotions only poorly; studies appeared to indicate that such people are more likely to develop rheumatoid arthritis. To describe the linkage he was seeing, and to name the field he was pioneering, Solomon coined the term psychoimmunology: the study of the mind-immune connection. But the medical world was not ready for him. The idea that personality—an individual's lifelong emotional and mental style—could bring on a failure of the immune system was just too radical for most medical professionals to accept.

Evidence of links between the immune system and the brain accumulated. In 1974 research psychologist Robert Ader of the University of Rochester in New York proved—quite serendipitously—that rats' immune systems could respond to something the animals learned. When a creature, whether animal or human, comes to associate one event with an unrelated occurrence, the result is called a conditioned response. The phenomenon was named by Russian psysiologist Ivan Pavlov, who trained dogs to salivate at the sound of a bell, an event unrelated to eating. He did this by repeatedly giving the animals tidbits of food and, each time, ringing the bell just when the sight and smell of the food made their mouths start to water. After sufficient repetitions, the dogs would salivate whenever Pavlov rang the bell, even though there was no food on hand.

In a similar type of experiment, Ader trained rats to dislike sweetened water by making them ill with a drug at the moment they tasted the water. By chance, the drug he had chosen was an immunosuppressant; as well as causing a stomachache, it damped down the workings of the immune system by halting the division of white blood cells. To his astonishment, Ader found that when the rats later tasted sweetened water without receiving the drug, they suppressed the production of antibodies as a conditioned, or learned, response. Medical theory offered no clue as to how this might occur, since the immune system was not known to be connected to the brain, the organ of learning. The discovery, wrote Ader, raised "innumerable issues concerning the normal operation and modifiability of the immune system." Could mental events besides conditioning affect the immune system? Could the normal operation of immunity include mental events?

Ader suspected that the nervous and endocrine (hormonal) systems provided communications links between the brain and the immune system. He therefore lengthened Solomon's word to psychoneuroimmunology and used it as the title for a book of papers he collected from other researchers working on topics that seemed to him to be related. That volume, published in 1981, became the first comprehensive reference in the budding field—which, for the sake of manageable pronunciation, came to be known as PNI.

Before long, a physician duplicated Ader's conditioning strategy with a human patient. Pediatrician Karen Olness was treating a 10-year-old girl named Marette, who was seriously ill with lupus. Anxious to minimize the unpleasant side effects of an immunosuppressive drug—the same one that Robert Ader gave to his rats—Olness taught Marette to associate the drug with two strong sensory experiences: the flavor of cod-liver oil and the scent of rose perfume. "We knew from research that taste and smell are most easily conditioned," Olness later explained. "We felt that by using both a taste and a smell, we might double our chances of success." After repeated associations with the immunosuppressant, the oil and perfume became conditioned stimuli, and Marette's body responded to them as if to the drug. "Over time," recounted Olness, "we gave Marette less of the drug than we would have given to a child who was not undergoing such conditioning, and Marette did equally well."

Conditioning can also work to produce episodes of ill health, as has been clearly shown in studies of asthma. Susceptibility to asthma attacks—a constriction of the respiratory tract

that brings on wheezing and chest tightness—is determined by a number of factors, including genetic predisposition, psychological stress, and exposure to allergens. Physicians have long known that the allergy factor lends itself to conditioning. For an asthmatic who is allergic to cat fur, the mere sight of a cat, even at a distance, may bring on an attack.

The discovery of the immune system's ability to learn conditioned responses, as well as the time-honored placebo effect, suggested to many medical researchers that PNI could have a bright future. But the black-box issue had not gone away. Until investigators could pry the lid off that metaphorical box—uncover ways in which the brain and immune system could communicate, not just indications that they did—progress was likely to be slow and hesitant.

As it happened, some of the anatomical and chemical underpinnings of such communication came to light at about the same time Ader discovered that the immune system is teachable. In the early 1970s, a multidisciplinary team of researchers—physiologist Hugo Besedovsky, immunologist Ernst Sorkin, and biochemist Adriana del Rey—placed electrodes in the brain of a rat, then stimulated the animal's immune system by injecting some foreign cells. After the

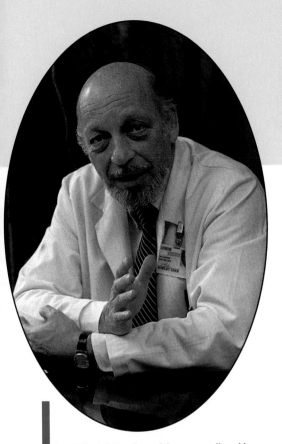

Dr. Robert Ader showed in a groundbreaking experiment with rats in 1974 that an animal's brain can influence its immune system. This tantalizing work formed the cornerstone of subsequent efforts by researchers to demonstrate that mental attitude can affect the outcome of disease.

injection, the electrical activity in the rat's brain increased—"the first clear indication that the brain actually knew what the immune system was doing," as Besedovsky said.

Later, a French immunologist by the name of Gerard Renoux, working from the brain down, destroyed portions of a mouse's cerebral cortex to see the effect on the immune system. He found that if he cut out part of the left side of the cortex, the production and efficiency of white blood cells dropped; if he excised part of the right side, those same cells became somewhat more aggressive. This suggested to him that, under normal circumstances, the left side stimulates the immune system, whereas the right side suppresses it. Renoux drew a sweeping conclusion: "The brain controls the immune system the same way it controls behavioral activities. There must be cooperation between the right and left sides."

The case for contact between the brain and the body's disease defenses became indisputable in the early 1980s when investigators began to find neural pathways to the immune system. Working with both animals and humans, Karen Bulloch of the State University of New York at Stony Brook spotted nerve fibers radiating from the brainstem and spinal cord into the tissues of the thymus, the gland where T cells mature and de-

velop the ability to distinguish "self" from "nonself." David Felten of the University of Rochester extended the search to the spleen—with similar results. "There," he said, "sitting in the middle of these vast fields of cells of the immune system, was a bunch of nerve fibers." Since then, he and other investigators have found neural fibers reaching to the bone marrow and the lymph nodes—to all the important sites of the immune system, in fact.

Meanwhile, another, quite different mode of communication between the brain and the immune system was found, this one involving chemical messengers that travel through the bloodstream and lymphatic system until they meet cells that have just the right molecular structures—docking points called receptors—to receive them. One of the leading hunters of these messengers is neuropharmacologist Candace Pert. She first came to the scientific world's attention as a graduate student at Johns Hopkins University in the early 1970s when, along with her supervisor Solomon Snyder, she found that the brain has special receptors for opiates such as morphine and heroin. This was startling, since the receptors apparently had some sort of use. (As Pert put it, "God presumably did not put an opiate receptor in our brains so we could eventually discover how to get high with opium.") An answer was soon forthcoming. It turned out that the body has its own natural opiates. Dubbed endorphins (for endogenous morphines), they are what joggers learned to thank for their feelings of well-being and euphoria after the first few miles.

The endorphins are only part of the body's vast array of natural pharmaceuticals. Pert has focused on neuropeptides, strings of amino acids that, in their role as neurotransmitters, flow from the brain to cells throughout the body; they may also flow from immune cells to the brain, since such cells also manufacture peptides. She and other researchers have now cataloged about 50 neuropeptides, which have specialized effects that range from causing a stinging pain in a fresh wound to telling the body that it is thirsty and must conserve what water it has. The immune system cells bearing neuropeptide receptors on their surfaces are monocytes and macrophages, the mature, battle-ready form of monocytes. In Pert's view, macrophages act like "mobile synapses." She and her collaborator Michael Ruff theorize that neuropeptides can latch onto macrophages and change the speed or direction of their movement

according to the defensive needs of the moment.

When Pert began mapping brain tissue to see where peptide receptors are concentrated, she found dense clusters in those areas of the brain associated with emotions—the hypothalamus, for example. Considered from an evolutionary standpoint, this did not seem surprising. As she explains, "Emotions are so important in terms of regulating behavior and regulating survival that the very first successful evolution in that direction would be preserved. After all, the great pleasures of life—eating and sex—are both necessary for survival, and there's tons of emotional wiring around those behaviors in humans." Since the neuropeptides carry information to and from the part of the brain that is concerned with emotional states, Pert calls the molecules the "biochemical units of emotion."

The chemical-message traffic between the immune system and the brain had turned out to be enormously complex. In 1979, for example, immunologist Edwin Blalock of the University of Alabama discovered that immune system cells can manufacture a variety of hormones—among them, ACTH (adrenocorticotropic hormone,

which stimulates activity in the adrenal gland), reproductive hormones, thyroid-stimulating hormone, and growth hormone. "Anything we looked for is there," he says. "It's as if the immune system is just a bunch of miniature, floating pituitary glands." He suggests that these hormones enable the immune system to coordinate its activities with the body's other systems. For example, as the immune system cells fight a disease, the secretion of thyroid-stimulating hormone could adjust the metabolism and heart rate.

To many researchers, discoveries such as these seemed to be a clarion call for new medical strategies—widened therapeutic campaigns that would take in body and mind at the same time. In spite of the apparent existence of various pathways between the brain and immune system, however, the medical establishment was still not ready to embrace the new connectivist ideas. The New England Journal of Medicine was a leader of the resistance. An article in the June 1985 issue concluded, on the basis of a study of patients in advanced stages of pancreatic, gastric, and lung cancer, that psychological and social factors did not influence recurrence rates or survival time. In the same issue, one editor declared, "It is time to acknowledge that our belief in disease as a direct reflection of mental

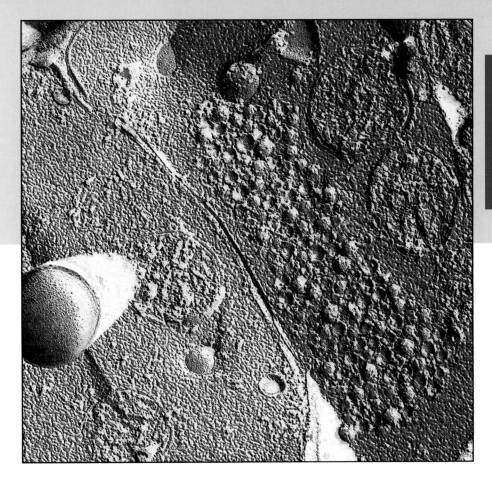

The diagonal channel in this electron micrograph is a synapse, the minuscule gap between one nerve cell and another. Just to the right of the gap is an area populated by pebble-shaped synaptic vesicles. These structures release neurotransmitters, the medium of communication between brain and body, including the immune system.

decreased levels of interferon and natural killer (NK) cells and heightened levels of epinephrine and norepinephrine. People enduring the long-term stress of taking care of a spouse with Alzheimer's disease had generally weakened immune functions and greater incidence of colds and other respiratory-tract infections. Similarly impaired immune functions occur in people suffering from clinical depression, bereavement, or the upheaval of divorce or separation. There is clear statistical evidence that the more bad events a person encounters in a given time period, the greater the risk for infectious illness.

The experience of stress turns out to be highly subjective, very much a matter of a person's point of view and interpretation. Not everyone reacts the same way to a given set of events: One person's overwhelming burden may be seen by someone else as a challenging work load or a pleasurable level of excitement. Says a researcher in the field, "People who feel in control of life can withstand an enormous amount of change and thrive on it. People who feel helpless can hardly cope at all."

PNI investigations show that a negative approach to life—expecting the

state is largely folklore." But the tide was inexorably turning, and within a few years the same journal was publishing studies documenting links between emotions and illness.

A number of these articles focused on stress and its possible effects on the immune system. The groundwork for the investigations had been laid as far back as World War I, when researchers identified a biochemical reaction to danger that they called the fight-or-flight response. When a person experiences fear or anger, the brain releases a flood of stress hormones, including epinephrine (also known as adrenaline). As a result, the heart beats faster, the blood pressure rises, and blood vessels dilate and contract selectively to divert blood

flow to the muscles, preparing them for emergency action. Digestion slows, and—as investigators later learned—so do immune functions, freeing all bodily resources for the all-out muscular exertion of fighting or fleeing. Such a reaction was invaluable in the danger-filled world of our evolutionary ancestors. But for most people in most present-day situations, neither fight nor flight is appropriate. Moreover, the response can be harmful if it operates continuously. Continual stress prolongs the body's state of fight-or-flight arousal; the body prepares for both and does neither, with damaging results. The blood pressure remains chronically high and the immune system chronically suppressed.

Researchers who studied various groups of people in stressful life situations found an array of disturbances in their immune system reactions. Medical students taking exams had

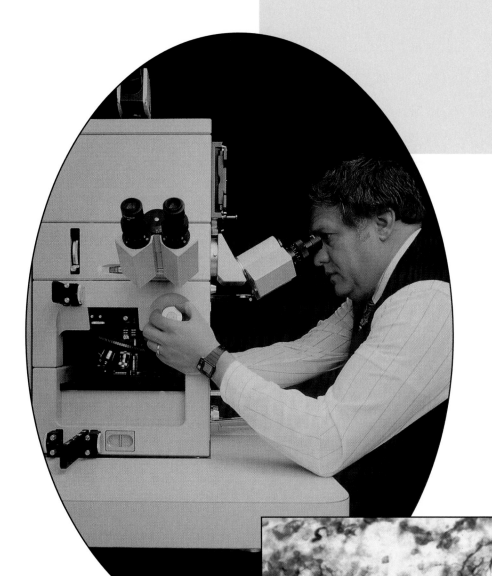

worst, expecting setbacks and defeats—interferes with immune functions; conversely, optimists have generally stronger immune system activity. In a study of 150 students carried out at the Virginia Polytechnic Institute and State University in the mid-1980s, psychologist Christopher Peterson determined that pessimists had twice as many infectious illnesses as optimists—and made twice as many visits to doctors. Another research project showed that optimists who undergo surgery recover faster than pessimists.

Optimism is closely related to the sense of hope, which often springs from the feeling of having control

Dr. David Felten peers into a sophisticated microscope that he and others used to find the terminus of nerve cells entering immune system organs. As shown in the image at right of a rat's spleen, neurons *(black threads)* lead not to vessels or other tissues in the organ, but to immune cells located there.

over events. Much evidence indicates that increased control, even on a small and personal scale, can reduce health problems. In a study in which nursing-home residents were accorded more control over their daily lives—the choice of whether to see a movie or not, for instance—they became happier and more active within weeks. They were also less prone to illness than companions who did not have those seemingly trivial choices, and 18 months later, those with greater control were more likely to be alive. AIDS patients, too, survive longer if they feel more in command of their lives and are more active.

Recent PNI studies have confirmed —with cell counts and chemical levels—the ancient wisdom that people need the comfort of friendships and a network of social support. Among medical students at exam time, for instance, those who described themselves as lonely had the least active natural killer cells. Marital status jibes with this finding: Single people are at a greater risk for depression and other health problems than people with spouses. Similarly, individuals who isolate themselves when they are ill tend to grow sicker. And in a study of cancer patients, psychological oncologist Sandra Levy of the University of Pittsburgh found that the more social support cancer patients felt they had, the greater the vigor of their NK cells.

Experts disagree over how much a negative, pessimistic outlook can be changed. Some researchers consider attitude toward life not a permanent personality trait but merely a habit that has been learned over time—a habit that, with perseverance, can be unlearned. Matthew Budd, director of behavioral medicine at Boston's Harvard Community Health Plan, speaks of "coaching" patients, helping them "shift the way they observe their 'realities' and see possibilities for new action." How they describe their lives is critically important, in his view, because "language generates reality." Christopher Peterson, who conducted the Virginia Polytechnic study, makes the same point, observing that what separates optimists from pessimists is their explanatory style. When accounting for setbacks or problems, optimists speak of things that are external, transitory, and specific. In talking about a missed promotion, for example, the optimist says that it was "just a bad break; maybe next time." But the pessimist, seeing the causes as internal, permanent, and all-encompassing, says, "I'm a poor excuse for a human being; I'll never succeed at anything important."

Such chronic passivity, which figures heavily in depression, is what Martin Seligman, director of clinical training at the University of Pennsylvania, calls learned helplessness—a behavioral style with marked physiological consequences, some of them involving the immune system. "States of mind, such as hope, have corresponding brain states," says Seligman. "Learned helplessness reaches down to the cellular level and makes the immune system more passive." In one study, people were made to feel helpless by a loud noise that kept them from concentrating on a puzzle. Afterward, their macrophages were moving sluggishly.

One of Seligman's key findings is that in any group of test subjects—animals or humans—about a third are innately optimistic and refuse to give in to helplessness. (Indeed, these may be the same one-third of subjects who respond positively to placebos—obtaining improvements largely because they confidently expect them.) But optimism need not be inborn; just as people have learned helplessness, says Seligman, they can learn optimism. One popular style of counseling, called cognitive therapy, trains patients to change the way they describe, think about, and react to events in their lives.

The training program in cognitive therapy is built around five basic elements. First, the patient is taught to pay attention to the so-called automatic thoughts that flit through the mind in times of depression; these fleeting thoughts are self-condemning and unchallenged explanations for the patient's plight. Second, the patient learns how to combat the thoughts with contrary evidence—facts that show the situation is not permanent or disastrous or proof of personal inadequacy. Third, the patient learns to find new explanations to replace the utterly negative, self-hating automatic thoughts. Fourth, the patient learns how to veer away from negative thoughts at times of pressure, putting off any self-analysis until a calmer moment. Finally, the patient learns to question assumptions that underlie the depression—such psychological traps as a belief that one is a failure unless universally liked, or that a perfect solution must be found for every problem.

As an example of the subtle but important changes that occur in the course of cognitive therapy, Seligman describes the case of a woman named Tanya, who entered therapy in a state of extreme depression, seeing her marriage as failing and her three children as uncontrollable. Her pessi-

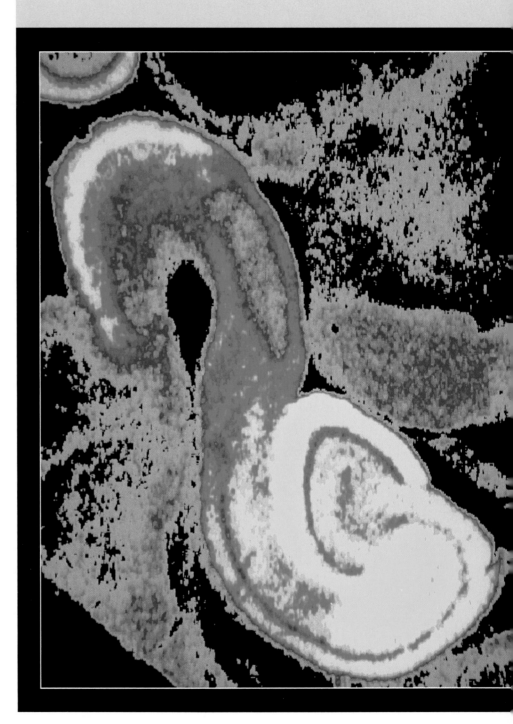

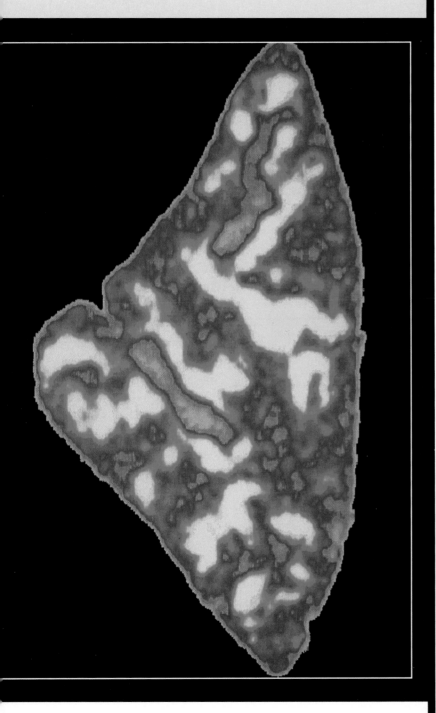

The Body's Own Essence of "Bliss"

In December 1992, after four years' trial and error in the lab, Dr. William Devane and a team of researchers at Hebrew University in Jerusalem succeeded in purifying a single drop of a new neurotransmitter from pig brains. The oily substance is chemically related to tetrahydrocannabinol (THC), the active ingredient in marijuana—a similarity that led Devane to name his discovery anandamide, from the Sanskrit for "bliss."

In addition to producing a sense of well-being in marijuana smokers, THC also reverses the effects of the eye disease glaucoma and may figure in such diverse ailments as Huntington's disease and pathological under- and overeating.

THC is also known to suppress the immune system. Locations of anandamide receptors suggest a nervous system link with the immune system in animals—and presumably in humans—not too different from that of epinephrine (*page* 117). For example, yellow and green areas in a guinea pig's limbic system (*far left*), a part of the brain involved in the fight-or-flight response, indicate the presence of many anandamide receptors. Similar concentrations also appear in animal spleens—a sample from a rat appears at left—one site where B cells mature into antibody-producing plasma cells.

mism and self-contempt were boundless. She explained that she was disgusted with herself "because I always yell at my kids and never apologize." She said that she had no hobbies "because I'm no good at anything." But gradually she began to develop a new explanatory style, acknowledging that her problems had external causes rather than arising from her total worthlessness, that they were specific, not all-pervading and all-destroying, and that they were not necessarily lasting. Her words of explanation continued to recognize difficulties in her life ("I had to go to church alone because my husband was being mean to me and wouldn't go"; "I run around looking like rags because the kids have to get their school clothes"), but they now allowed for the possibility of change. She could take action to deal with the problems. Her depression began to lift.

The hope of many researchers, of course, is that when people replace their bleak views of the present and future with more positive views, the shift may bolster the immune system's fight against many disease processes, possibly including cancerous tumors. Seeking evidence of such an effect, in the late 1980s Martin Seligman and the University of Pittsburgh's Sandra Levy provided 12 weekly cognitive-therapy sessions to patients with melanoma and colon cancer, helping them to recognize, interrupt, and change their negative ways of thinking about their situations. Analysis of their immune system functions showed that the natural killer cell activity was much greater than in patients who got no cognitive therapy.

One team of researchers has investigated what the expression of strong emotions does to the immune system. They asked a group of actors to improvise a performance evincing deep sadness, then to dramatize great joy. When the actors were immersed in intense feelings, their blood was checked for immune-cell changes. In the light of other PNI findings, the researchers were not surprised to see that the joyful emotions resulted in a boost to the immune system. What startled them was that giving expression to sadness did the same thing. In 1988 other researchers found similar effects in people who had experienced traumatic events and later spent time—just 20 minutes a day, four days in a row—writing about them. The writing process brought painful feelings to the surface of the mind. It was an unpleasant experience but brought a payoff of enhanced immune-cell activity.

Bottling up emotions, then, appears to add to the body's burden of stress and can be hazardous to health. In many people, unreleased psychological distress finds an outlet in physical ailments. The American Medical Association has reported that two-thirds of all visits to doctors are for complaints that are not diseases; instead, the ailments are physical manifestations of stress. In medical parlance, such patients are somatizers: That is, they translate psychological anguish into bodily symptoms, sometimes highly symbolic. In one striking case, an aspiring violinist had to drop out of music school because persistent eczema kept her hand red and raw. After a psychotherapist helped her explore her feelings toward her family, she realized she felt guilty about not staying home to care for her elderly grandmother. Once the emotions were in the open, the eczema cleared up, and the student returned to her studies. In another case, a young mother, exhausted from her firstborn's colicky restlessness and her husband's increasing withdrawal, developed a severe rash just under her wedding band—though it was not the only gold ring she wore. The third finger of her left hand became so swollen that she had to have the wedding ring cut off, as if saying with her body what she had never said out loud, that she wished she had not married.

Some researchers have come to the conclusion that habitually bottled-up emotions and continual frustration of the fight-or-flight response might lead to cancer. Psychologist Lydia Temoshok has postulated a correlation between the occurrence of cancerous tumors and an extremely passive response to stress that she calls Type C behavior. The term is an echo of the Type A and Type B nomenclature invented in connection with some heart disease studies in the 1960s. Type A people, according to this descriptive system, are highly competitive, anxious, self-centered, and given to angry outbursts. They are more susceptible to heart attacks and strokes at an early age, as their habitual hostility takes a toll on their cardiovascular systems. People with a so-called Type B coping style have a generally more relaxed, laid-back approach; they express emotions appropriately and take steps to meet their own needs as well as those of others. They can shrug off the petty irritations of the day, and they enjoy better cardiovascular health.

In the early 1990s, Temoshok added Type C to the list, describing it as a "disease-prone" coping style at the opposite end of the behavioral

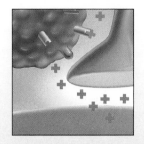

A Dialogue of Consequence

Chemical communication between the brain and the immune system seems to travel both ways. When the immune system signals the brain, the goal is to enhance the body's infection-fighting abilities, or so it is thought. For example, when macrophages in the bloodstream produce a molecule of the regulatory substance interleukin-1 (IL-1), it has the same effect when it reaches the brain as IL-1 synthesized in the brain itself: It causes the nervous system to promote sleep and raise body temperature, both helping the immune system fight bacteria.

If the brain contacts the immune system, however, the result can be to restrain the body's defenses. Such is the case whenever the body's fight-or-flight response is kindled. The purpose of slowing the immune system to near idle, of course, is to divert energy that would be used to fight infection toward helping the body survive the more immediate threat. (Unfortunately, the fight-or-flight response is triggered not only by a mugger in the dark but also by chronically stressful circumstances of modern life that can be neither escaped nor overcome. Suppression of the immune system because of long-term stress can thus ultimately promote disease.)

The brain has two ways of throttling the immune system, both mediated by the hypothalamus. In one, chemicals called hormones, traveling throughout the body by way of the bloodstream, are the agents of immune system suppression. In a more recently discovered process, signals travel along nerve cells directly to organs of the immune system, carried there by chemicals called neurotransmitters. Both routes are explained on the following pages, using as examples the hormone cortisol, a product of the adrenal glands, and the neurotransmitter epinephrine.

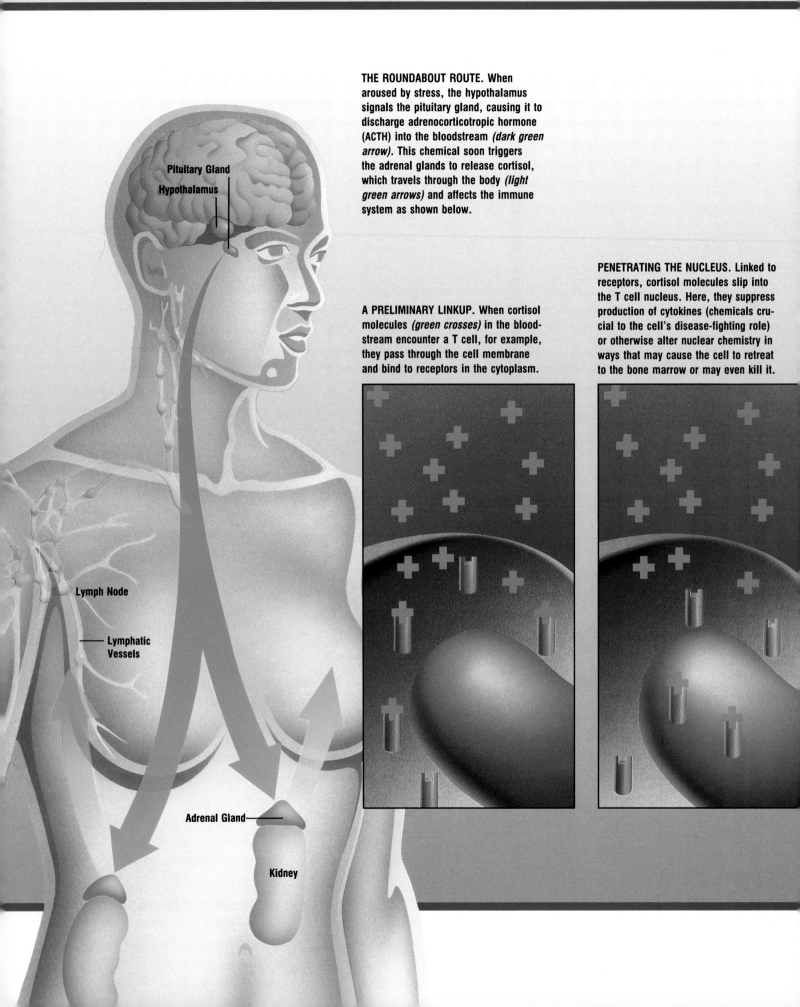

THE ROUNDABOUT ROUTE. When aroused by stress, the hypothalamus signals the pituitary gland, causing it to discharge adrenocorticotropic hormone (ACTH) into the bloodstream *(dark green arrow)*. This chemical soon triggers the adrenal glands to release cortisol, which travels through the body *(light green arrows)* and affects the immune system as shown below.

Pituitary Gland

Hypothalamus

Lymph Node

Lymphatic Vessels

Adrenal Gland

Kidney

A PRELIMINARY LINKUP. When cortisol molecules *(green crosses)* in the bloodstream encounter a T cell, for example, they pass through the cell membrane and bind to receptors in the cytoplasm.

PENETRATING THE NUCLEUS. Linked to receptors, cortisol molecules slip into the T cell nucleus. Here, they suppress production of cytokines (chemicals crucial to the cell's disease-fighting role) or otherwise alter nuclear chemistry in ways that may cause the cell to retreat to the bone marrow or may even kill it.

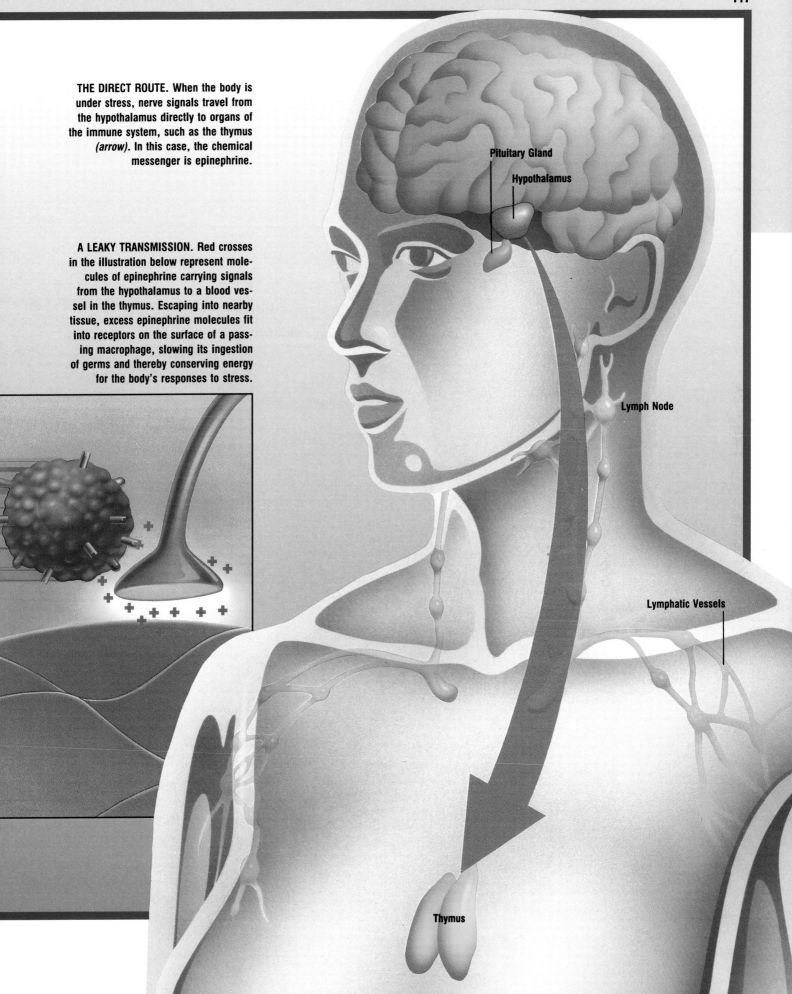

THE DIRECT ROUTE. When the body is under stress, nerve signals travel from the hypothalamus directly to organs of the immune system, such as the thymus *(arrow)*. In this case, the chemical messenger is epinephrine.

A LEAKY TRANSMISSION. Red crosses in the illustration below represent molecules of epinephrine carrying signals from the hypothalamus to a blood vessel in the thymus. Escaping into nearby tissue, excess epinephrine molecules fit into receptors on the surface of a passing macrophage, slowing its ingestion of germs and thereby conserving energy for the body's responses to stress.

Pituitary Gland

Hypothalamus

Lymph Node

Lymphatic Vessels

Thymus

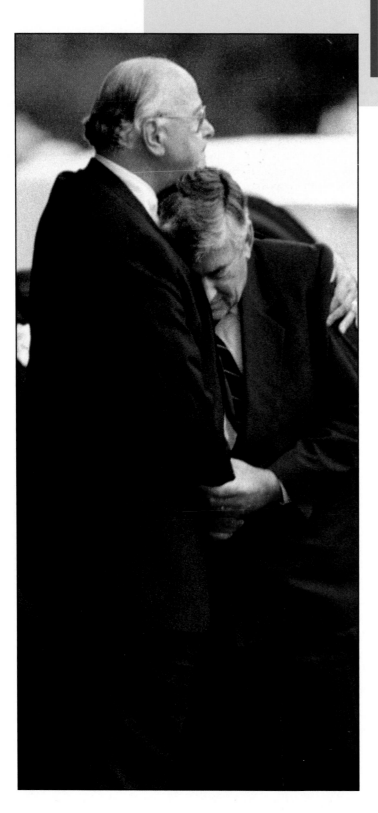

Assailed by grief, veteran stock-car driver Bobby Allison leans on a friend at the funeral for his son Davey, killed in a helicopter crash. Venting the profound sadness experienced at the death of a loved one is believed to assist the immune system in recovering from the initial, weakening shock of such an experience.

spectrum from the aggressive Type A. Type C copers are passive and depressed, with angry and hostile feelings that they don't express. Eager to please others, they have little sense of control in their lives, and little awareness of their own feelings or needs. In fact, they share many traits with George Solomon's "rheumatoid personality"; they are quiet and introverted, reliable and conscientious, conforming and self-sacrificing. This personality profile appears to invite immune system problems.

Temoshok speculates that a Type C individual is emotionally numb because of increased levels of endorphins, the body's natural morphine-like painkiller. Constant burying of emotions may produce a flood of painkillers, which may in turn suppress the immune system and make the Type C coper more susceptible to disease. Type C coping—which Temoshok also calls the repressor personality—has been linked to arthritis and may also bring on asthma and high blood pressure.

A causative link to cancer has been suggested by some animal studies showing that injected tumor cells are more likely to thrive in distressed, passive, defeated animals—those who behave like Type C people. One carefully designed experiment yielding such results was conducted in 1982 by nurse Madelon Visintainer, working with Martin Seligman at the University of Pennsylvania. First, she implanted in each rat a precisely calibrated number of cells of a sarcoma that, if not fought off by the immune system, is invariably fatal. Previous trials had determined that the number of tumor cells in the implants would, under normal circumstances, produce a 50 percent mortality rate.

Visintainer then divided the rats into three groups. One group was subjected to mild electric shocks but was given the power to shut off the shocks by pressing a bar. The second group received the same mild shocks but was given no opportunity to escape them. The third group was not shocked at all. Within a month, the implanted cancer cells took quite different tolls in the three groups. The normal mortality ratio prevailed among the rats that received no shocks: Half lived and half died. Among the rats who were able to control the situation by switching off the electric shocks, 70 percent rejected the tumor cells and lived. Among the helpless rats, only 27 percent fought off the cancer; 73 percent succumbed to the disease.

Most experimenters decline to extrapolate from such evidence to humans, because the tumors in the animal studies are from injected foreign cells and do not mirror the origins and onset of cancer in people. As for human studies, there is still no hard evidence that people with Type C traits get cancer more often than any other population group. And if Type C coping style and cancer do turn up together disproportionately, perhaps the explanation is that patients have responded to the depressing diagnosis of cancer with emotional withdrawal and stoicism. Temoshok nonetheless remains convinced that Type C coping puts people at risk for cancer. On the bright side, she says that, since Type C is a learned coping behavior, it can be unlearned and replaced with a healthier, more open way of dealing with emotions—what she calls a "hardy" coping style of expressing feelings and releasing them. The key, she says, is to "contact your feelings, soften your defenses, and change your relationships."

While the notion that coping style can be a risk factor for cancer is controversial and unproved, there is considerable evidence that mood can affect the progression of the disease once it has appeared. Cancer patients seldom die from their first tumor.

What kills is metastasis—the spread of the cancer into other parts of the body. This is done by individual cancer cells that move into the lymphatic system and bloodstream, making their way to new locations, where they divide and become a new tumor.

The immune system's defense against these colonizers is its floating arsenal of natural killer cells, designed to intercept the enemy cells as they migrate to new tissue. "We can treat primary tumors," notes John Hiserodt, former head of the Pittsburgh Cancer Institute Immunology Program. "We can cut them out, we can melt them down with chemotherapy agents, but patients may still die of metastases." Therefore, for cancer patients, he says, "the NK cells may be the most important thing that enables them to live." Since so many studies suggest that the number and activity of NK cells is affected by the patient's state of mind, Lydia Temoshok observes that, for cancer researchers, "the question should no longer be, 'Can our bodies effectively wipe out cancer,' but 'Why don't our bodies effectively wipe out cancer?'"

To promote sturdy immune system defenses, holistic-minded healthcare providers employ an array of tools in addition to cognitive therapy. Among the options are relaxation, meditation, biofeedback, hypnosis, and imagery. Each one involves a kind of purpose-

Relaxation and the Immune Response

Since stress caused by the fight-or-flight response dampens the powers of the immune system (*pages* 115-117), it stands to reason that consciously relieving stress might help restore the body's defenses to full strength. And research has shown that even a brief respite can indeed have this useful effect.

The goal of unwinding is to invoke the body's relaxation response, characterized chiefly by decreases in heart and breathing rates. According to one prominent theory, relaxing affects the limbic system, the region of the brain linked to the emotions and to involuntary functions such as digestion. The limbic system, in turn, may signal the hypothalamus to send neurotransmitters through the nerves or hormones through the blood that reverse changes brought on by stress. For example, it might undo a stress-related rise in cortisol levels with a message to cut back on cortisol production or to make a hormone that counters cortisol's effects.

There are many roads to the relaxation response. Some of them involve soothing the body by touch of one kind or another. The oil treatment shown at right traces its origins to a Hindu rite of purification dating from ancient times. Massage, whether performed as acupressure or a similar discipline from Asia, or administered in the more vigorous Swedish style (*far right*), also has a positive impact on the immune system.

Eliciting the relaxation response can be a solitary exercise as simple as breathing deeply for 20 to 25 minutes while consciously relaxing every muscle, one at a time, from toes to head. Hypnotism also works. A trainer is advisable at first, but most individuals can soon learn to hypnotize themselves. The same is true of biofeedback, wherein people learn to raise or lower muscle tension, heartbeat, and even body temperature. Initially, specialized electronic gear monitors and reports the levels of such factors with a rising or falling tone or a line on a computer screen (*page* 122), but most people are quickly weaned from the equipment.

ful attention. In meditation, for example, the purpose is to quiet the mind, often by paying attention to breathing. According to one teacher of the practice, meditators experience a dramatic drop in anxiety and a new, calmer consciousness of their body.

Biofeedback makes use of electrical equipment to convey to patients certain information about their body—their muscle tension, for example, or skin temperature, pulse, breathing, or sweating. This electronically aided self-awareness can help control such disorders as headaches, high

blood pressure, anxiety, and chronic pain, and many patients find biofeedback a useful tool in learning how to achieve a state of relaxation.

Hypnosis induces a relaxed state in which the mind becomes open to suggestion. Typically, a therapist will lead patients into hypnosis by words alone, instructing them to relax and focus their attention. Patients may also learn self-hypnosis and can make

suggestions to themselves while in the receptive state. In either case, hypnosis is often not classified as a trance, as popular belief would have it; rather, many researchers view it as a condition of intense and focused concentration, with full awareness of the surroundings. Precisely what is happening in the brain in the hypnotic state remains uncertain and much debated, but there is considerable evidence of bodily responses to suggestions. Hypnosis has been used to trigger or suppress poison-ivy allergic reactions and outbreaks of herpes-

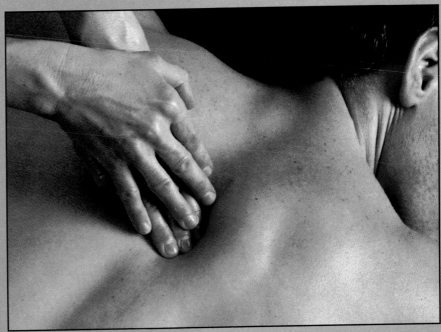

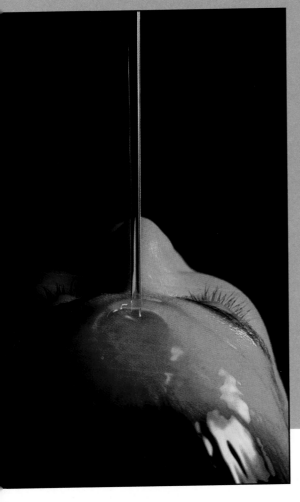

SHIRODHARA DRIP. Warm, herb-infused oil flows onto the forehead in a technique borrowed from Ayurveda, which means "science of life" in Sanskrit. Devotees claim that this source of relaxation also helps the body rid the blood of harmful toxins.

MASSAGE. Rubbing and kneading the body is one of the oldest of all healing techniques. Prolonged massage, besides easing tension, has been found to not only increase the number of natural killer (NK) cells in the body but improve their effectiveness as well.

virus. It has served to reduce the severity of asthma attacks and control anxiety or the fear of pain. Some studies indicate that it can also affect immune system responses.

Imagery is a type of therapy in which patients learn to relax and mentally picture the functioning of their bodies, either directly or metaphorically. In one example of direct imagery, an asthma patient was told to spend 20 minutes, twice a day, envisioning his lung passages opening so that air would move through easily; the exercise reduced the severity and frequency of attacks. Metaphorical imagery can take many forms. Nick Hall, a PNI specialist at the University of South Florida, found that when cancer patients systematically imagined a state of war against cancer cells—a war waged with bullets or spears or combat aircraft, for instance —their lymphocytes multiplied and fought tumors more successfully. Some patients are reluctant to create such militaristic images, but the destruction of cancer cells can be visualized in other ways. Psychological oncologist Wendy Schan of the Memorial Cancer Institute in Long Beach, California, has reported good physical responses after patients take on their cancers with nonbellicose images; a typical example might be pulling weeds out of a garden.

The use of these behavioral inter-

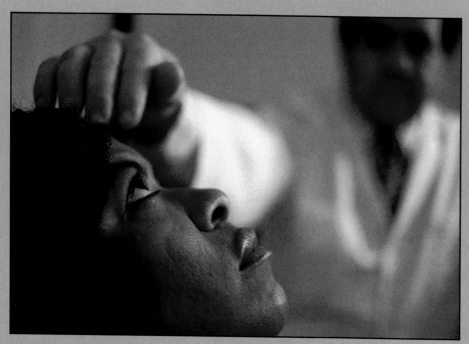

HYPNOSIS. A woman enters a state of deep relaxation by concentrating intently on a voice, an object, or a mental image. Delivered under hypnosis, suggestions to focus on the immune system can have an effect. In one study, children increased their production of immunoglobulins, which fight disease-causing organisms.

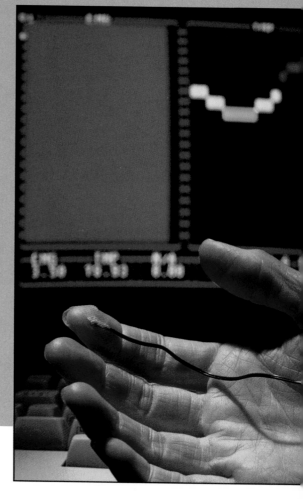

BIOFEEDBACK. A sensor taped to a finger detects changes in heart rate, which a computer displays as a graph. By concentrating on making the trace rise or fall, a person can learn to lower heart rate for increased relaxation.

ventions is no longer limited to a lonely handful of mavericks practicing them in defiance of the medical establishment: The largest of cancer-care centers—including Sloan Kettering in New York, Johns Hopkins in Baltimore, and Georgetown Hospital in Washington, D.C.—now offer support groups where patients can learn stress-management techniques and receive psychological counseling, and this sort of expanded care is spreading rapidly. Information about new

modes of treatment and promising lines of research is being disseminated more efficiently than ever. In the mid-1980s the National Institutes of Health (NIH)—the United States' flagship medical-research center—established the Behavioral Immunology Committee to review funding for research on AIDS and to help scientists

from different fields to pool information. By opening avenues of communication among the various biomedical disciplines, the committee aims to prevent a recurrence of the situation of the early 1960s, when immunologists worked in isolation, unaware of what psychologists, neurologists, and other scientists were doing.

In October 1992, NIH set up an Office of Alternative Medicine (OAM). Its mission, spelled out by the U.S. Congress, is to investigate methods and techniques previously untested and unapproved by the medical mainstream and to determine what is effective. On the list for scrutiny: traditional and ethnic healing practices; structural manipulations such as chiropractic and massage; mind-body control techniques such as counseling, guided imagery, and relaxation; diet and other lifestyle changes. The purview of the OAM will also embrace some little-known electromagnetic therapies and such exotic pharmacological strategies as using bee pollen to treat asthma and combating tumors with shark cartilage or compounds synthesized from human urine. In every study OAM supports, a required ingredient will be collaboration between a mainstream scientist who is expert in standard research procedures and an alternative practitioner highly experienced with the healing method under examination.

Given the official interest in exploring all therapeutic possibilities and the increasing cross-fertilization among medical disciplines, there is every reason to expect that medicine in the future will be an enlarged realm. Some prognosticators antici-

pate the routine use of psychology to prevent and treat physical diseases. "We'll see much greater emphasis on prevention," predicts Martin Seligman, who expects psychology will become "much more useful to well people. Right now, most individuals don't benefit from psychological intervention until they become mentally disturbed"—which often means they are plagued with physical health problems. Seligman's recent work includes a program in Philadelphia to teach children "the techniques of learned optimism. My goal is to protect them against depression and poor health in adulthood." Jonas Salk, who developed the polio vaccine, agrees with this approach. If he were just starting out in medicine now, he has said, "I would still do immunization, but it would be psychological rather than biological." There could hardly be a more resonant endorsement of the mind-body connection than that.

In the same way that many medical researchers are working to develop innovative treatments grounded in a new partnership with the immune system, many physicians expect to develop new relationships with their patients—on terms that will undoubtedly call upon the patient's resources at least as much as on the physician's. David Felten, a discoverer of

neural pathways between the brain and the immune system, believes that the doctor of tomorrow will not act as "the initiator or provider of healing in a passive patient" but instead will become "a participant in healing." Just as immunologists have learned to talk to psychologists—and the immune system has been communicating with the central nervous system all along—so doctors and patients are learning to team up in cooperative relationships.

Candace Pert has described a recurring dream in which she faces the chasm that divides the old ways of practicing medicine from the new. "There's a guy on the other side who is telling me to jump," she said, "and I'm scared to jump." In her waking hours, however, Pert and her colleagues have already done a great deal to move medicine across that chasm to an arena where the mind is in and of the body, and where the emotions play a recognized role in physical illness and health. Looking forward to such an enlightened future, Pert has another prediction: "It's going to be so quickly forgotten," she says, "how controversial this all was."

DETECTING RENEGADES: THE IMMUNE SYSTEM AND CANCER

Cancer is a disease of disorder. The illness is usually caused when environmental triggers—anything from smoking to sunlight—act on certain susceptible genes in a way that turns them into anarchists. Deserting the elegant precision of the body's cellular design, the cancerous cells cease serving their host and regress to a primitive form whose only aim is its own reproduction.

Unless the body's defenses can stop them, the renegade cells proliferate chaotically and clump together to form tumors. If they are malignant, the tumors invade nearby tissues, block their functions, and steal their nutrients, thereby killing them. Moreover, the tumors can send out colonists that travel through blood or lymphatic fluid to establish new tumors far removed in the body from the original, or primary, mass. Once this process, called metastasis, occurs, the cancer becomes extremely hard to treat and usually poses a mortal threat.

Cancer cells are among the greatest challenges that can confront the immune system because, though primitive in form, they are amazingly sophisticated in function. They are adept at camouflage, for example. The warped progeny of the body's own cells, they may not wave the obvious antigen flags that alert the immune system to such invaders as viruses and bacteria. They travel under the passport of "self," not "other."

Even so, rebellious cells may give off subtle signs that act as a call to arms for immunity's defending troops. For example, cancer cells may have surface irregularities that brand them as foreign, or they may have too few or too many normal cell markers, signaling danger to immune cells. The picture at right shows a defending killer lymphocyte wedged between two tumor cells. If, after inspecting the cells' surfaces, the defender recognizes them as cancer, it will assault them with an injection of lethal chemicals.

Categorized according to the type of tissue in which they arise, there are more than 100 different types of cancer, including cancers of the immune system itself. All are dangerous, but researchers are making headway against them. Some of the newest therapies, still experimental, harness the immune system's own ability to seek and destroy wayward cells.

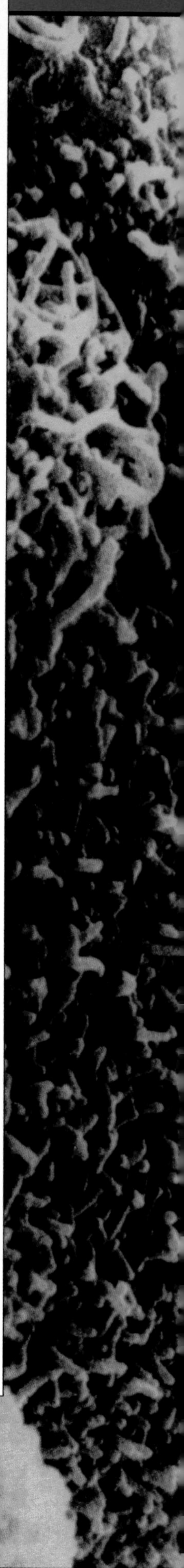

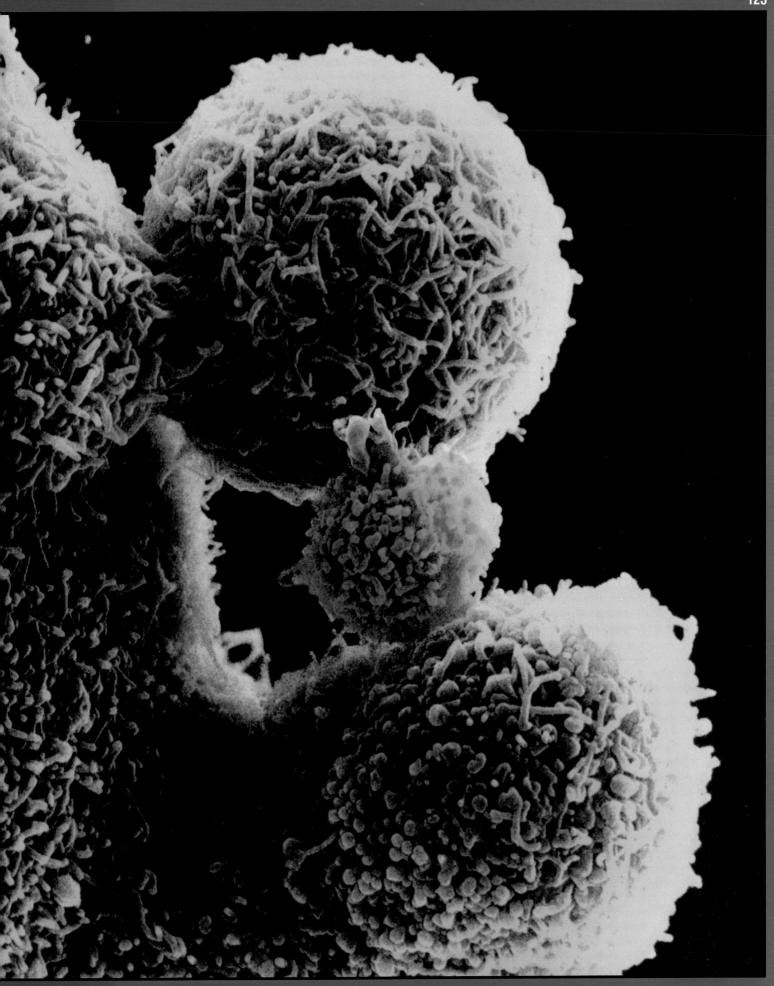

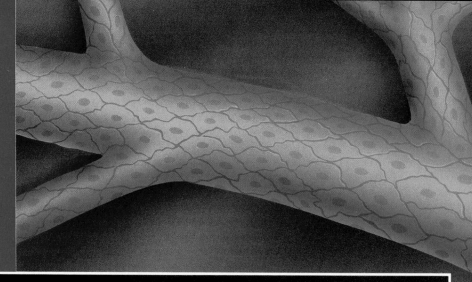

A CELL TURNS TRAITOR

Most cells are team players. They perform specific jobs, working under rules that unite them as organs such as the liver or the skin. Cancer starts when one cell abandons its team loyalties and strikes out on its own disorderly course.

Although a cell may go awry simply through random mutation, the trouble more commonly starts with a gene that is predisposed to turn the cell cancerous. These genes, called proto-oncogenes, are normally suppressed. However, they can be switched on by any factor that alters the cell's DNA —environmental triggers that include radiation, pollutants, certain viruses, certain hormones, and harmful compounds in foods or in tobacco smoke. Generally, exposure to more than one agent is required before DNA is damaged enough for a cell to turn traitor. The type of cancer that arises depends on which type of cell goes bad.

Once activated, the proto-oncogene transforms its host into a cancerous cell that, unchecked, has the potential for endless replication. Replication does not always happen, however. The bad cell may repair itself, or it may die or fail to reproduce, thus removing any threat of cancer. If it does reproduce, the eventual result is a tumor, one that invades surrounding tissues and may then begin the aggressive and complex assault of metastasis depicted here.

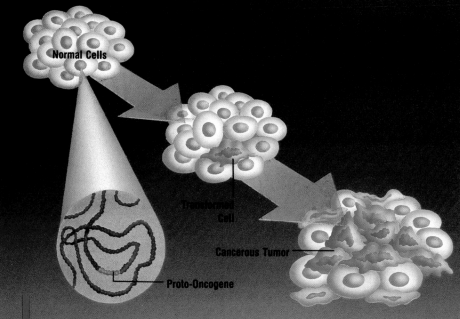

Normal Cells

Transformed Cell

Cancerous Tumor

Proto-Oncogene

From the clump of normal cells shown above, a portion of one cell's DNA strand has been highlighted. The DNA contains a proto-oncogene *(orange)*. In its normal state, this gene is probably helpful to the cell, contributing to its growth and function. Awakened by a trigger, however, the proto-oncogene becomes an oncogene—a cancer gene —and it starts making proteins that cause the cell to become cancerous, as seen in the second stage. The cell changes form, abandons its normal function, and grows and divides uncontrollably. In the third stage, the cancer cells, multiplying out of control, have formed a tumor, pushing aside the normal cells and causing them to die off.

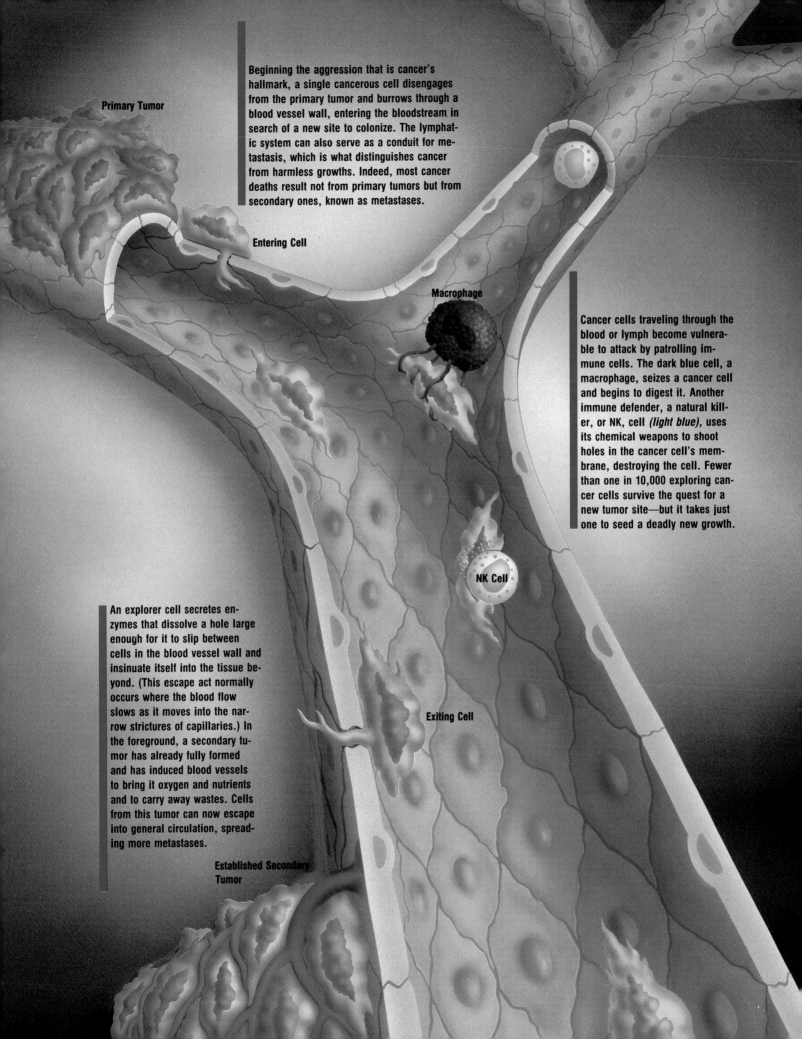

Primary Tumor

Beginning the aggression that is cancer's hallmark, a single cancerous cell disengages from the primary tumor and burrows through a blood vessel wall, entering the bloodstream in search of a new site to colonize. The lymphatic system can also serve as a conduit for metastasis, which is what distinguishes cancer from harmless growths. Indeed, most cancer deaths result not from primary tumors but from secondary ones, known as metastases.

Entering Cell

Macrophage

Cancer cells traveling through the blood or lymph become vulnerable to attack by patrolling immune cells. The dark blue cell, a macrophage, seizes a cancer cell and begins to digest it. Another immune defender, a natural killer, or NK, cell *(light blue)*, uses its chemical weapons to shoot holes in the cancer cell's membrane, destroying the cell. Fewer than one in 10,000 exploring cancer cells survive the quest for a new tumor site—but it takes just one to seed a deadly new growth.

NK Cell

An explorer cell secretes enzymes that dissolve a hole large enough for it to slip between cells in the blood vessel wall and insinuate itself into the tissue beyond. (This escape act normally occurs where the blood flow slows as it moves into the narrow strictures of capillaries.) In the foreground, a secondary tumor has already fully formed and has induced blood vessels to bring it oxygen and nutrients and to carry away wastes. Cells from this tumor can now escape into general circulation, spreading more metastases.

Exiting Cell

Established Secondary Tumor

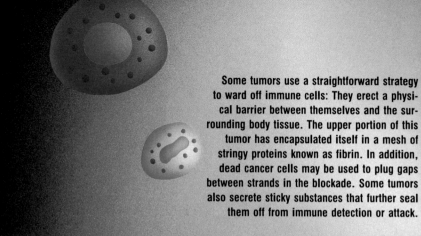

EVADING THE IMMUNE ASSAULT

Despite its drastic inner transformations, a cancer cell may present a surface that appears nearly normal to immune cells. When it is effective, this camouflage allows renegade cells to sneak by defenders undetected. Even when cancer cells display antigens that should mark them for destruction—as they often do—immune cells may encounter a tumor only to hold fire and even retreat. In many cases, cancerous tumors removed from patients have been found to contain cytotoxic, or killer, T cells that seem to be completely inactive.

Scientists have several theories about how cancer cells manage to escape attack. One hypothesis is that the surfaces of the traitor cells confuse the defenders by rapid changes, appearing at times normal, at times not. Another theory suggests that cancer cells simply shed the cancer-specific antigens that would otherwise target the cells themselves for destruction. The immune system's antibodies attach themselves to these free-floating decoys, allowing the real culprits to pass unmolested.

Researchers have found that tumors can secrete substances that block immune cells or that render them inactive. The secretions may even prevent the immune cells from reproducing or cause them to kill themselves or one another. However, the exact mechanisms of these and other tumor defenses are not yet well understood.

Some tumors use a straightforward strategy to ward off immune cells: They erect a physical barrier between themselves and the surrounding body tissue. The upper portion of this tumor has encapsulated itself in a mesh of stringy proteins known as fibrin. In addition, dead cancer cells may be used to plug gaps between strands in the blockade. Some tumors also secrete sticky substances that further seal them off from immune detection or attack.

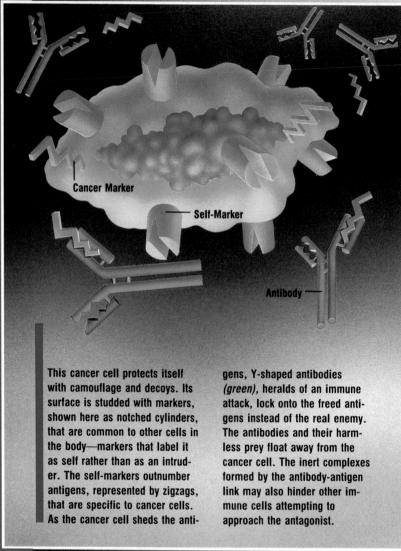

This cancer cell protects itself with camouflage and decoys. Its surface is studded with markers, shown here as notched cylinders, that are common to other cells in the body—markers that label it as self rather than as an intruder. The self-markers outnumber antigens, represented by zigzags, that are specific to cancer cells. As the cancer cell sheds the antigens, Y-shaped antibodies (green), heralds of an immune attack, lock onto the freed antigens instead of the real enemy. The antibodies and their harmless prey float away from the cancer cell. The inert complexes formed by the antibody-antigen link may also hinder other immune cells attempting to approach the antagonist.

Healthy cells use chemicals to communicate. In a process largely a mystery to scientists, cancer cells emit the same messages but with a different effect: the thwarting of the immune system. Here the tumor discharges chemicals (orange crosses) that neutralize or kill incoming immune cells. A helper T cell tries to send an alarm (purple crosses) to a killer T cell, but the message is blocked. The tumor's chemicals have signaled a macrophage (far right) to leave the scene, while a neutrophil (lower right) has died from the tumor's toxins.

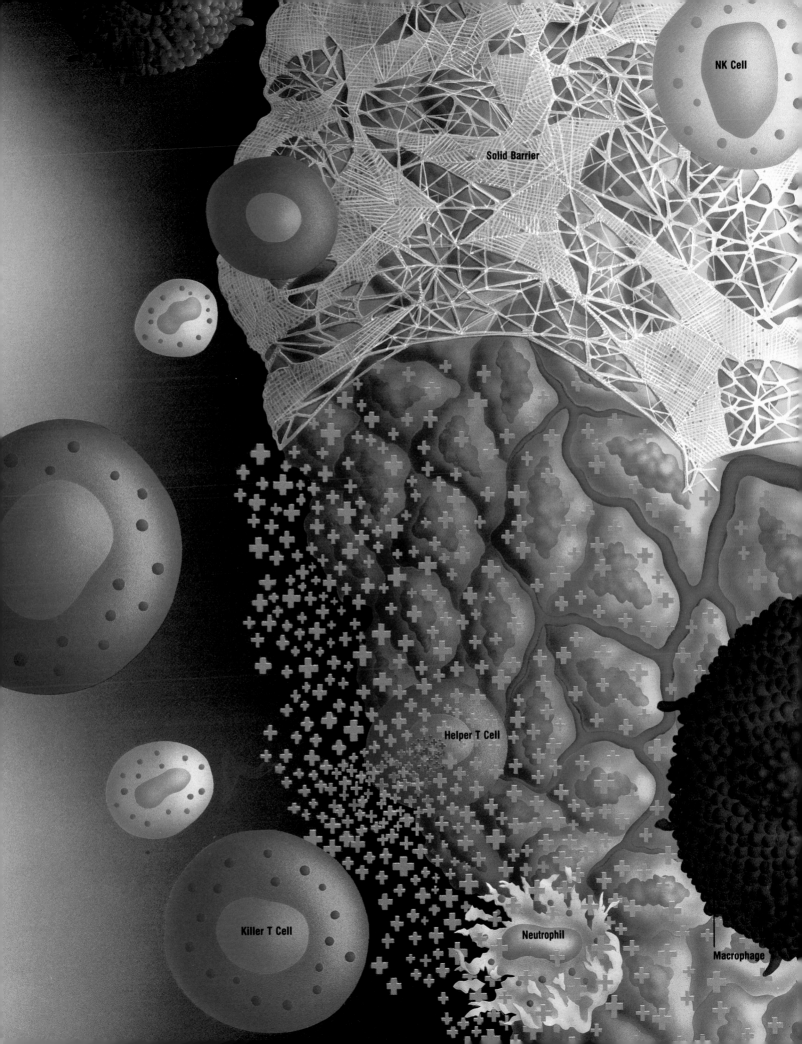

OLD ENEMY, NEW WEAPONS

Doctors stock their anticancer arsenal with three conventional weapons: surgery, radiation, and chemotherapy drugs. They usually administer these treatments in combination, first excising tumors, then applying radiation or chemotherapy, or both, to kill any stray cancer cells. This orthodox approach works best when the cancer is detected early—before a primary tumor metastasizes.

New armaments are being tested, however, and some may prove to be highly effective even after metastasis. There are, for instance, substances known as biological response modifiers, or biologicals for short. These are the innumerable chemicals produced by the immune system itself to regulate its many functions. In tests, laboratory-produced biologicals seem able to help boost the immune response. They also appear to have some cancer-killing properties of their own. Immune chemicals such as interferons, interleukin-2 (IL-2), and tumor necrosis factor (TNF) are now being used in conjunction with more traditional therapies.

Some new therapies, such as those detailed at right, are designed to make the immune response itself the primary weapon. Thus far their testing on humans has been limited to last-resort treatment for patients near death. Years of trials lie ahead to determine whether their benefits outweigh any risks they might pose.

Antibodies Take Aim

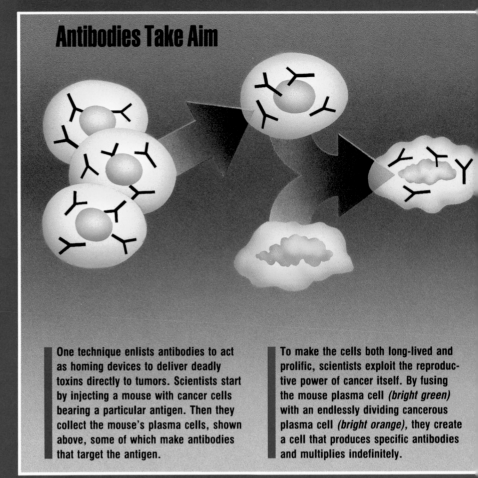

One technique enlists antibodies to act as homing devices to deliver deadly toxins directly to tumors. Scientists start by injecting a mouse with cancer cells bearing a particular antigen. Then they collect the mouse's plasma cells, shown above, some of which make antibodies that target the antigen.

To make the cells both long-lived and prolific, scientists exploit the reproductive power of cancer itself. By fusing the mouse plasma cell *(bright green)* with an endlessly dividing cancerous plasma cell *(bright orange)*, they create a cell that produces specific antibodies and multiplies indefinitely.

Boosting the Body's Own Killers

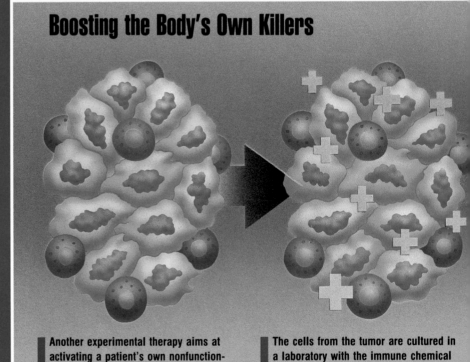

Another experimental therapy aims at activating a patient's own nonfunctioning T cells—those apparently stymied by tumors—into effective cancer killers. Physicians excise a tumor containing both cancer cells *(orange)* and killer T cells *(purple)* that have gathered at the site of the cancer.

The cells from the tumor are cultured in a laboratory with the immune chemical interleukin-2, or IL-2, represented here by gray crosses. The IL-2 stimulates the T cells to grow and multiply rapidly.

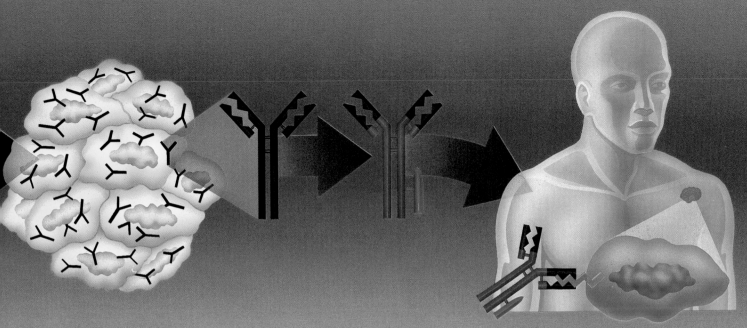

The fused cells grow and divide. To extract from them the most effective antibodies, researchers must separate the cells, start a new colony from each one, and then test antibodies culled from each colony. The prize—the antibody that matches the cancer antigen most closely—forms the basis for therapy.

For use in humans, the mouse antibody is often replaced with human proteins *(dark green)* to reduce the odds that the patient will have an immune reaction to the mouse proteins. The antibody is then armed with a potent toxin or a radioactive molecule *(red)*.

Finally, the armed antibody is injected into a cancer patient. The antibody should home in on cancer cells bearing the corresponding antigen and—with minimal damage to surrounding healthy cells—kill the cancer cells with the chemical missiles or radiation.

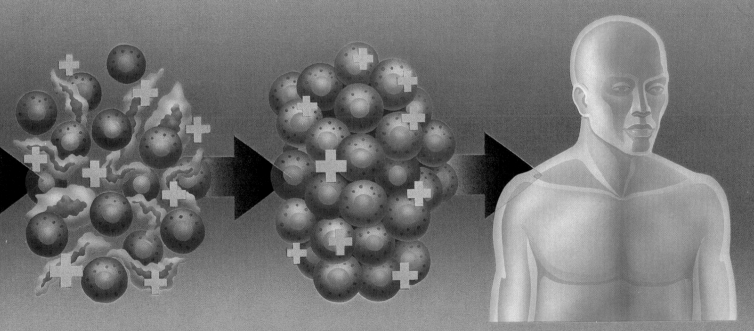

Bolstered by IL-2, the T cells aggressively attack the cancer cells. Along with stimulating the growth and reproduction of T cells, IL-2 sends out signals that help the passive T cells recognize and assault the enemy. (Some immune chemicals may also be themselves toxic to cancer.)

After 30 to 45 days of incubation, the T cells have destroyed all the cancer cells. Primed by more IL-2, they have proliferated into a powerful army of cancer-cell assassins.

Some 200 billion activated T cells are injected intravenously into the patient, along with an extra dose of IL-2. In theory, the pumped-up T cells will attack all familiar-looking cancer cells. And as the T cells are long-lived and can create memory cells, they should confer immunity to similar future tumors.

A KILLER T CELL TRIUMPHANT

A fully functioning killer T cell has just destroyed a cancer cell, reducing it to harmless debris. Once a killer T cell has made contact with its target, it secretes powerful proteins that puncture the cancer cell's outer membrane. As the cancer cell's fluids leak out, the cell disintegrates, a method of execution known as lysis. Little is left of the cancer cell but its smooth round nucleus *(far right)* and the remains of its internal structures, which look like bubbles spilling away from the nucleus. Ruffles stand up on the surface of the T cell, indicating that it is ready to enter another battle.

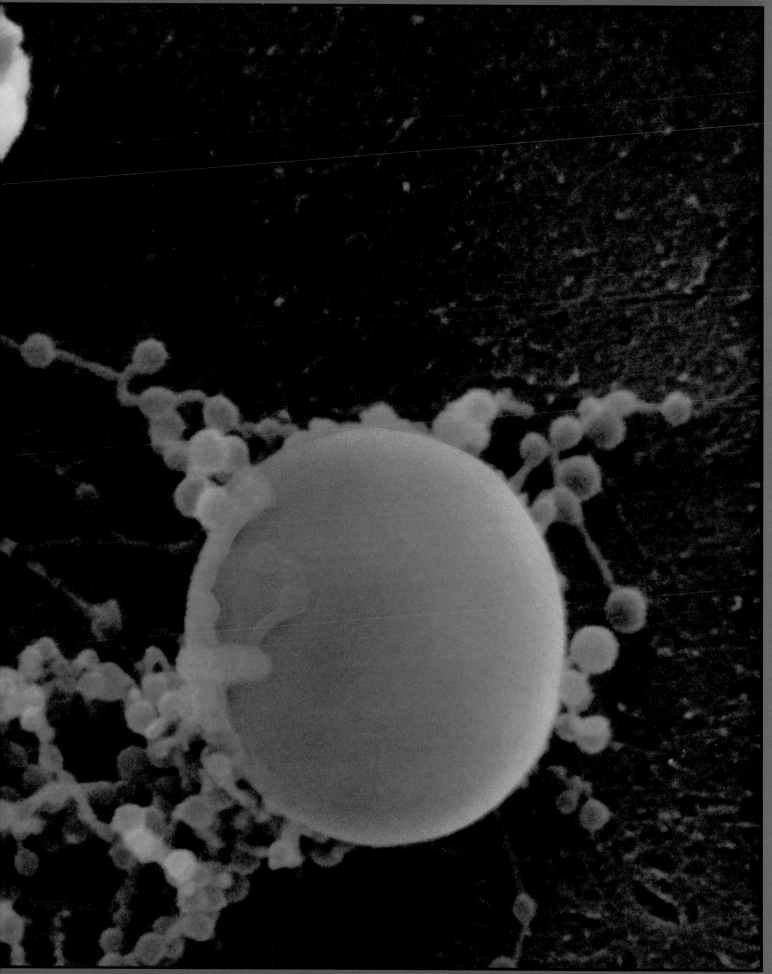

GLOSSARY

Acquired immunodeficiency syndrome (AIDS): an affliction caused by the human immunodeficiency virus (HIV), which attacks helper T cells; the virus destroys the immune system's ability to fend off disease.

Allergen: an apparently harmless antigen, such as pollen, that can trigger an inappropriate immune response in susceptible people.

Antibiotic: a chemical substance that is detrimental to bacteria and other microorganisms.

Antibody: protein, produced by B cells, whose job it is to combine with an antigen and thereby mark it for destruction.

Antigen: any substance that can provoke an immune response.

Autoimmune disease: a disorder resulting from an immune system attack against the body's own normal tissues.

Bacteria: one-celled organisms, some of which can cause infections.

Basophil: a type of white blood cell that participates in immune and allergic reactions.

B cell: one of a class of lymphocytes that mature into antibody-producing plasma cells.

Blood serum: the clear, pale-yellow liquid component of blood, separate from blood cells and clotting factors. *See also* Plasma.

Bone marrow: soft tissue at the center of bones. Red bone marrow is the fundamental production site for all blood cells.

Cilia: filamentary extensions of the surface of a cell. In humans, cilia help clean debris from the respiratory tract and other passages.

Complement: special proteins in the blood that assist antibodies in ridding the body of antigens and that contribute to inflammation.

Cytokine: any of several types of chemi-

cals, produced by various immune cells, that serve as messengers to facilitate the immune response.

Cytotoxic T cell: a type of immune cell that recognizes antigens on target cells and attacks and destroys them; also known as a killer T cell.

Endorphin: any of a class of molecules, produced naturally in the brain and in other tissues, that bind to the brain's opiate receptors; endorphins thus can act as painkillers and can induce a euphoric state of mind.

Enzyme: a type of protein that serves as a catalyst for a specific function.

Eosinophil: one of a class of white blood cells important in the immune response to parasitic infections.

Epinephrine: a stress-related hormone that increases heart rate, blood pressure, and carbohydrate metabolism; also known as adrenaline.

Epithelium: cellular tissue covering surfaces or lining cavities.

Granulocyte: a class of white blood cells with granules in their cytoplasm that contain destructive chemicals. The three types of granulocytes are basophils, eosinophils, and neutrophils.

Helper T cell: a T cell that alerts B cells to begin the process of antibody production. Helper T cells can release interleukin, which stimulates other T cells.

Histamine: a chemical released by mast cells during allergic reactions that causes inflammation.

Hormone: a chemical, released by glands and a few other organs, that travels through the bloodstream and regulates the activities of specific tissues, organs, and other glands. Some hormones help fight infection by regulating the immune system.

Human immunodeficiency virus (HIV): the

retrovirus that causes AIDS. *See also* Acquired immunodeficiency syndrome.

Hypothalamus: a structure in the brain that controls autonomic functions, such as body temperature, and also produces hormones and neurotransmitters.

Immunodeficiency disease: any condition that results from an inadequate immune response.

Immunoglobulin (Ig): one of several classes of protein molecules that function as antibodies.

Infection: invasion of the body by organisms that cause disease or injury to tissue.

Inflammation: a reaction of tissues to injury or infection, usually characterized by redness, pain, swelling, heat, and impaired function. Inflammation may be a by-product of the immune system's response.

Interferon: any of three antiviral proteins produced by certain white blood cells and by cells that have been invaded by viruses.

Interleukin: one of several types of cytokines, secreted by certain cells of the immune system, that have various stimulating effects on the immune response of other cells.

Killer T cell: *See* Cytotoxic T cell.

Lupus: any of several autoimmune disorders that involve inflammation of connective tissue.

Lymph: a clear fluid that contains white blood cells and is carried in the vessels of the lymphatic system.

Lymphatic system: the network of lymph nodes and vessels that—together with such lymphoid organs and tissues as the spleen, the thymus, and red bone marrow—produce and transport white blood cells.

Lymph nodes: tissue masses located throughout the body that contain immune cells and serve as filters for antigens in the blood and lymph.

Lymphocyte: the general term for white blood cells produced in the lymphatic system and lymphoid tissues. Lymphocytes include B cells, T cells, and natural killer cells.

Lymphokine: a nonantibody product of lymphocytes that can have destructive or stimulating effects on other cells.

Lysozyme: an enzyme present in tears, mucus, and other body fluids that protects against bacteria.

Macrophage: a large, mature phagocyte that can ingest and destroy invading microbes, foreign particles, cancerous or diseased cells, and cellular debris. Macrophages, which need no direction from the immune system to act, can also alert lymphocytes to the presence of antigens and produce a variety of cytokines.

Major histocompatibility complex (MHC): genes that produce a group of proteins that mark an individual's cells as self.

Mast cell: a type of cell related to basophils and found in the skin, tongue, lungs, and linings of the nose and intestine. Mast cells produce histamine.

Memory cell: a long-lived lymphocyte—either a T cell or a B cell—that retains the ability to recognize a specific antigen and can respond rapidly to second or subsequent attacks.

Monocyte: a circulating phagocyte that ingests microbes, invading particles, and cellular debris. Monocytes mature into macrophages.

Myelin: a white fatty substance that insulates the axons of many neurons.

Natural killer (NK) cell: a type of lymphocyte that attacks and kills virus-infected cells or cancer cells without direction from any other part of the immune system.

Neuropeptide: any of various peptides found in neuronal tissue that either serve as neurotransmitters or affect the action of neurotransmitters.

Neurotransmitter: any of a number of chemical substances, synthesized by neurons, that are involved in the transmission of electrochemical impulses across the synaptic gap from one neuron to another or from a neuron to a muscle or gland.

Neutrophil: one of the three types of granulocytes; involved in inflammation and other immune responses.

Pathogen: a disease-causing substance or organism.

Peptide: a compound consisting of two or more amino acids linked in a specific way.

Phagocyte: a white blood cell that can engulf and destroy pathogens, foreign particles, and cellular debris. *See also* Macrophage; Monocyte.

Placebo: an inert substance assumed by a patient to be a medicine.

Plasma: the fluid part of blood, after removal of red and white cells; plasma devoid of clotting factors is known as serum.

Plasma cell: an antibody-producing cell that derives from a B cell.

Platelets: cell fragments in the blood that play an essential role in blood clotting and wound repair. Platelets can also activate certain immune defenses.

Pseudopod: a temporary extension of the cytoplasm of a cell. Macrophages use pseudopods to engulf debris or invading microorganisms.

Receptor: a protein molecule on the surface of a cell to which complementary molecules, such as neurotransmitters or antigens, can bind.

Retrovirus: a type of virus, such as the one responsible for AIDS, that contains RNA rather than DNA. Instead of simply inserting its genetic material into the DNA of a host cell, as conventional viruses do, retroviruses must first convert their RNA into DNA.

Rheumatoid arthritis: an autoimmune disease in which inflammation occurs in the joints.

Spleen: a lymphoid organ in the abdomen that serves as a filter for blood, a production site for antibodies, and the body's major place for the dismantling of worn red blood cells.

Stem cell: a cell in red bone marrow that generates any of several specialized blood cells.

Suppressor T cell: a T cell that can inhibit the actions of B cells and other T cells when the threat of infection is over. Many scientists question their existence and speculate that some T cells simply kill other T cells.

T cell: one of several types of lymphocytes that are key players in the immune response. *See also* Cytotoxic T cell; Helper T cell; Suppressor T cell.

Thymus: a lymphoid organ in the chest where T cells mature.

Toxin: poison that is produced by an organism, such as the bacterial toxin that causes tetanus.

Vaccine: a preparation containing a killed or weakened form of a disease-causing agent, such as bacteria, used to stimulate the production of antibodies and the development of immunity.

Vacuole: a cavity, surrounded by its own membrane, inside a cell.

Virus: a pathogenic microorganism that consists of DNA or RNA and various enzymes, all surrounded by a protein coat; viruses reproduce by invading living cells and using cellular mechanisms to create multiple copies of themselves.

White blood cell: any of a group of nearly colorless immune cells, including lymphocytes, granulocytes, and phagocytes.

BIBLIOGRAPHY

BOOKS

ABC's of the Human Body. Pleasantville, N.Y.: Reader's Digest, 1987.

Ader, Robert, David L. Felten, and Nicholas Cohen (eds.). Psychoneuroimmunology (2d ed.). San Diego: Academic Press, 1991.

Alberts, Bruce, et al. Molecular Biology of the Cell (2d ed.). New York: Garland Publishing, 1989.

Berg, Paul, and Maxine Singer. Dealing with Genes. Mill Valley, Calif.: University Science Books, 1992.

Bessis, Marcel. Corpuscles: Atlas of Red Blood Cell Shapes. New York: Springer-Verlag, 1974.

Borysenko, Joan. Minding the Body, Mending the Mind. Reading, Mass.: Addison-Wesley, 1987.

Clayman, Charles B. (ed.). The American Medical Association Encyclopedia of Medicine. New York: Random House, 1989.

Considine, Douglas M., and Glenn D. Considine. Van Nostrand's Scientific Encyclopedia (7th ed.). New York: Van Nostrand Reinhold, 1989.

Cotran, Ramzi S., Vinay Kumar, and Stanley L. Robbins. Robbins Pathologic Basis of Disease (4th ed.). Philadelphia: W. B. Saunders, 1989.

Davis, Joel. Defending the Body: Unraveling the Mysteries of Immunology. New York: Macmillan, 1989.

De Kruif, Paul. Microbe Hunters. New York: Harcourt, Brace & World, 1953.

Desowitz, Robert S. The Thorn in the Starfish. New York: W. W. Norton, 1987.

Dienstfrey, Harris. Where the Mind Meets the Body. New York: Harper Perennial, 1991.

Dowling, Harry F. Fighting Infection. Cambridge, Mass.: Harvard University Press, 1977.

Dreher, Henry. Your Defense against Cancer. New York: Harper & Row, 1988.

Dwyer, John M. The Body at War. New York: New American Library, 1988.

Fighting Cancer (Library of Health series). Alexandria, Va.: Time-Life Books, 1981.

Fleischer, B., and H. O. Sjögren. Superantigens. Berlin: Springer-Verlag, 1991.

Gallo, Robert C. Virus Hunting. New York: BasicBooks, 1991.

Gazzaniga, Michael S. Mind Matters. Boston: Houghton Mifflin, 1988.

Glasser, Ronald J. The Body Is the Hero. New York: Random House, 1976.

Goleman, Daniel, and Joel Gurin (eds.). Mind Body Medicine. New York: Consumer Reports Books, 1993.

Golub, Edward S., and Douglas R. Green. Immunology: A Synthesis (2d ed.). Sunderland, Mass.: Sinauer Associates, 1991.

Good, Robert A. (ed.). Immunobiology. Stamford, Conn.: Sinauer Associates, 1971.

Grollman, Sigmund. The Human Body: Its Structure and Physiology (4th ed.). New York: Macmillan, 1978.

Haggard, Howard W. Devils, Drugs, and Doctors. New York: Blue Ribbon Books, 1929.

Hensyl, William R. (ed.). Stedman's Medical Dictionary (25th ed.). Baltimore: Williams & Wilkins, 1990.

Hurley, Thomas J., III. "Placebos and Healing: A New Look at the 'Sugar Pill.'" In Noetic Sciences Collection, 1980-1990: Ten Years of Consciousness Research, ed. by Barbara McNeill and Carol Guion. Sausalito, Calif.: Noetic Sciences Institute, 1991.

Immune Power. Emmaus, Pa.: Rodale Press, 1989.

The Incredible Machine. Washington, D.C.: National Geographic Society, 1992.

Joklik, Wolfgang K., et al. (eds.). Zinsser Microbiology (20th ed.). Norwalk, Conn., 1992.

Joneja, Janice M. Vickerstaff. Understanding Allergy, Sensitivity, and Immunity. New Brunswick, N.J.: Rutgers University Press, 1990.

Justice, Blair. Who Gets Sick. Los Angeles: Jeremy P. Tarcher, 1988.

Kalat, James W. Biological Psychology (4th ed.). Pacific Grove, Calif.: Brooks/Cole, 1992.

Kemeny, M. E., et al. "Psychoneuroimmunology." In Neuroendocrinology, ed. by C. B. Nemeroff. Boca Raton, Fla.: CRC Press, 1992.

Kessel, Richard G., and Randy H. Kardon. Tissues and Organs: A Text-Atlas of Scanning Electron Microscopy. San Francisco: W. H. Freeman, 1979.

Kimball, John W. Introduction to Immunology (2d ed.). New York: Macmillan, 1986.

Kuby, Janis. Immunology. New York: W. H. Freeman, 1992.

Kushner, Irving (ed.). Understanding Arthritis. New York: Charles Scribner's Sons, 1984.

Lechtenberg, Richard. Multiple Sclerosis Fact Book. Philadelphia: F. A. Davis, 1988.

Levine, Arnold J. Viruses. New York: Scientific American Library, 1992.

Levy, Sandra M. Behavior and Cancer. San Francisco: Jossey-Bass, 1985.

Lewin, Benjamin. Genes IV. Oxford: Oxford University Press, 1990.

Lichtenstein, Lawrence M., and Anthony S. Fauci. Current Therapy in Allergy, Immunology, and Rheumatology (4th ed.). St. Louis: Mosby-Year Book, 1992.

McCabe, Philip M., et al. (eds.). Stress, Coping and Disease. Hillsdale, N.J.: Lawrence Erlbaum, 1991.

Macfarlane, Gwyn. Alexander Fleming. Cambridge, Mass.: Harvard University Press, 1984.

McGraw-Hill Encyclopedia of Science & Technology (6th ed.). New York: McGraw-Hill, 1987.

Mizel, Steven B. In Self-Defense. San Diego: Harcourt Brace Jovanovich, 1985.

Moyers, Bill. Healing and the Mind. New York: Doubleday, 1993.

Mudge-Grout, Christine L. Immunologic Disorders. St. Louis: Mosby-Year Book, 1992.

Nilsson, Lennart:
  The Body Victorious. London: Faber and Faber, 1985.
  A Child Is Born. New York: Delacorte

Press/Seymour Lawrence, 1990.

Paul, William E. *Immunology: Recognition and Response*. New York: W. H. Freeman, 1991.

Playfair, J. H. L. *Immunology at a Glance*. Oxford: Blackwell Scientific, 1987.

Powers of Healing (Mysteries of the Unknown series). Alexandria, Va.: Time-Life Books, 1989.

Professional Guide to Diseases (4th ed.). Springhouse, Pa.: Springhouse, 1992.

Roitt, Ivan M. *Essential Immunology* (6th ed.). Oxford: Blackwell Scientific, 1988.

Roitt, Ivan M., Jonathan Brostoff, and David K. Male. *Immunology* (3d ed.). St. Louis: Mosby, 1993.

Rose, Noel R., and Diane E. Griffin. "Virus-Induced Autoimmunity." From *Molecular Autoimmunity*, ed. by Norman Talal. UK: Academic Press, 1991.

Scott, Andrew. *Pirates of the Cell: The Story of Viruses from Molecule to Microbe*. Oxford: Basil Blackwell, 1985.

Seligman, Martin E. P. *Learned Optimism*. New York: Alfred A. Knopf, 1991.

Shurkin, Joel N. *The Invisible Fire*. New York: G. P. Putnam's Sons, 1979.

Silverstein, Arthur M. *A History of Immunology*. San Diego: Academic Press, 1989.

Singer, Maxine, and Paul Berg. *Genes & Genomes*. Mill Valley, Calif.: University Science Books, 1991.

Stites, Daniel P., and Abba I. Terr. *Basic and Clinical Immunology* (7th ed.). Norwalk, Conn.: Appleton & Lange, 1991.

Tauber, Alfred I., and Leon Chernyak. *Metchnikoff and the Origins of Immunology*. New York: Oxford University Press, 1991.

Temoshok, Lydia, and Henry Dreher. *The Type C Connection*. New York: Random House, 1992.

Tortora, Gerard J., and Sandra Reynolds Grabowski. *Principles of Anatomy and Physiology* (7th ed.). New York: HarperCollins, 1993.

Varmus, Harold, and Robert A. Weinberg. *Genes and the Biology of Cancer*. New York:

Scientific American Library, 1993.

Watson, James D., et al. *Molecular Biology of the Gene* (Vol. 1, 4th ed.). Menlo Park, Calif.: Benjamin/Cummings, 1987.

Weiner, Michael A. *Maximum Immunity*. Boston: Houghton Mifflin, 1986.

Weiss, Leon. *The Cells and Tissues of the Immune System*. Englewood Cliffs, N.J., 1972.

Wilson, David. *Body and Antibody* (4th ed.). New York: Alfred A. Knopf, 1972.

PERIODICALS

"AIDS Research Shifts to Immunity." *Science*, July 10, 1992.

Anderson, John A. "Allergic Reactions to Drugs and Biological Agents." JAMA, Nov. 25, 1992.

Angell, Marcia. "Disease as a Reflection of the Psyche." *New England Journal of Medicine*, June 13, 1985.

Angier, Natalie:
"Advance Seen in Finding 'Magic Bullet' for Cancer." *New York Times*, July 9, 1993.
"Discovery of Tumor Antigen May Point to Cancer Vaccine." *New York Times*, Nov. 5, 1991.
"Tumors May Suppress Immune Cells that Fight Cancer, Study Finds." *New York Times*, Dec. 11, 1992.

"AZT-Resistant HIV Seen." *Science News*, Mar. 18, 1989.

Barinaga, Marcia. "Pot, Heroin Unlock New Areas for Neuroscience." *Science*, Dec. 18, 1992.

Beardsley, Tim:
"Cross Reaction." *Scientific American*, Dec. 1991.
"Positive Response." *Scientific American*, Aug. 1991.

Besedovsky, Hugo O., Adriana E. del Rey, and Ernst Sorkin. "What Do the Immune System and the Brain Know about Each Other?" *Immunology Today*, 1983, Vol. 4, no. 12, pages 342-346.

"A Big Leap Forward in AIDS Research." *U.S. News & World Report*, Nov. 26, 1990.

Boon, Thierry. "Teaching the Immune Sys-

tem to Fight Cancer." *Scientific American*, Mar. 1993.

"The Bubble Boy's Lost Battle." *Time*, Mar. 5, 1984.

"Bubble Boy's Secret." *Time*, Apr. 19, 1993.

Budd, Matthew A. "New Possibilities for the Practice of Medicine." *Advances: The Journal of Mind-Body Health*, Winter 1992.

Bylinsky, Gene. "New Weapons against AIDS." *Fortune*, Nov. 30, 1992.

Caldwell, Mark. "The Immune Challenge." *Discover*, Dec. 1991.

Cassileth, Barrie R., et al. "Psychosocial Correlates of Survival in Advanced Malignant Disease." *New England Journal of Medicine*, June 13, 1985.

Clowe, John Lee. "The Changing World of AIDS." *Vital Speeches of the Day*, Dec. 15, 1992.

Cohen, Irun R. "The Self, the World and Autoimmunity." *Scientific American*, Apr. 1988.

Cohen, Sheldon, David A. J. Tyrrell, and Andrew P. Smith. "Psychological Stress and Susceptibility to the Common Cold." Reprinted from *New England Journal of Medicine*, Aug. 29, 1991.

Creticos, Peter S. "Immunotherapy with Allergens." JAMA, Nov. 25, 1992.

"The Defences." *Economist*, Aug. 1, 1992.

Demaret, Kent, and "Carol Ann." "David's Story." *People*, Oct. 29, 1984.

Diamond, Jared. "Nature's Infinite Book: The Mysterious Origin of AIDS." *Natural History*, Sept. 1992.

"Emerging from the Bubble." *Time*, Feb. 20, 1984.

Essex, Max, and Phyllis J. Kanki. "The Origins of the AIDS Virus." *Scientific American*, Oct. 1988.

Ezzell, Carol:
"AIDS: Immune System Infighting?" *Science News*, Nov. 23, 1991.
"Two Strides Toward a Workable AIDS Vaccine." *Science News*, Dec. 19/26, 1992.

Fackelmann, Kathy A.:
"Marijuana and the Brain." *Science News*,

Feb. 6, 1993.

"MS Researchers Find Missing Immune Link." *Science News*, Feb. 10, 1990.

"Myelin on the Mend." *Science News*, Apr. 7, 1990.

Fineberg, Harvey V. "The Social Dimensions of AIDS." *Scientific American*, Oct. 1988.

Gallo, Robert C., and Luc Montagnier. "AIDS in 1988." *Scientific American*, Oct. 1988.

Garelik, Glenn. "Chilling Events on a Tropical Isle." *Discover*, May 1985.

Gavzer, Bernard. "What Keeps Me Alive." *Parade Magazine*, Jan. 31, 1993.

Gorman, Christine. "Are Some People Immune to AIDS?" *Time*, Mar. 22, 1993.

Hall, Nicholas R. S., and Allan L. Goldstein. "Thinking Well." *The Sciences*, Mar. 1986.

Hall, Nicholas R. S., and Maureen P. O'Grady. "Regulation of Pituitary Peptides by the Immune System." PNEI, 1989, Vol. 2, no. 1, pages 4-10.

Hall, Stephen S. "A Molecular Code Links Emotions, Mind and Health." *Smithsonian*, June 1989.

Haseltine, William A., and Flossie Wong-Staal. "The Molecular Biology of the AIDS Virus." *Scientific American*, Oct. 1988.

Hellman, Caroline J. C., et al. "A Study of the Effectiveness of Two Group Behavioral Medicine Interventions for Patients with Psychosomatic Complaints." *Behavioral Medicine*, Winter 1990.

Henig, Robin Marantz. "Dr. Anderson's Gene Machine." *New York Times Magazine*, Mar. 31, 1991.

Herberman, Ronald B. "Tumor Immunology." *JAMA*, Nov. 25, 1992.

Herberman, Ronald B., and John R. Ortaldo. "Natural Killer Cells: Their Role in Defenses against Disease." *Science*, Oct. 2, 1981.

Heyward, William L., and James W. Curran. "The Epidemiology of AIDS in the U.S." *Scientific American*, Oct. 1988.

Hilchey, Tim. "Researchers Find Genetic Defect that Causes Rare Immune Disease." *New York Times*, Apr. 9, 1993.

Hooper, Judith. "Unconventional Cancer Treatments." *Omni*, Feb./Mar. 1993.

Horan, Richard F., Lynda C. Schneider, and Albert L. Sheffer. "Allergic Skin Disorders and Mastocytosis." *JAMA*, Nov. 25, 1992.

"How the AIDS Virus Attacks." *U.S. News & World Report*, Dec. 10, 1990.

Jamner, Larry D., Gary E. Schwartz, and Hoyle Leigh. "The Relationship between Repressive and Defensive Coping Styles and Monocyte, Eosinophile, and Serum Glucose Levels." *Psychosomatic Medicine*, 1988, Vol. 50, pages 567-575.

Jaret, Peter. "Our Immune System: The Wars Within." *National Geographic*, June 1986.

Jaroff, Leon:

"Giant Step for Gene Therapy." *Time*, Sept. 24, 1990.

"Stop That Germ!" *Time*, May 23, 1988.

Kaliner, Michael, and Robert Lemanske. "Rhinitis and Asthma." *JAMA*, Nov. 25, 1992.

Kelleher, Colm. "Beyond HIV: Assembling the AIDS Puzzle." *Omni*, June 1993.

Kiecolt-Glaser, Janice. "Psychoneuroimmunolgy: Can Psychological Interventions Modulate Immunity?" *Journal of Consulting and Clinical Psychology*, 1992, Vol. 60, no. 4, pages 569-575.

Kirkpatrick, R. A. "Witchcraft and Lupus Erythematosus." *JAMA*, May 15, 1981.

Koffler, David. "Systemic Lupus Erythematosus." *Scientific American*, July 1980.

Kolata, Gina:

"Limits Seen for Cancer Treatment that Was Hailed as Breakthrough." *New York Times*, May 8, 1990.

"Tests Show Infection by AIDS Virus Affects Greater Share of Cells." *New York Times*, Jan. 5, 1993.

"Lethal Cascade." *Scientific American*, Mar.

1993.

Levy, Sandra M., et al. "Prognostic Risk Assessment in Primary Breast Cancer by Behavioral and Immunological Parameters." *Health Psychology*, 1985, Vol. 4, no. 2, pages 99-113.

Lightfoot, Marjorie J. "The Art of Healing, the Science of Drama: How Acting May Affect the Immune System." *Advances: The Journal of Mind-Body Health*, Fall 1992.

Liotta, Lance A. "Cancer Cell Invasion and Metastasis." *Scientific American*, Feb. 1992.

"Living with Your Self." *Scientific American*, Nov. 1988.

Lockey, Richard F. "Future Trends in Allergy and Immunology." *JAMA*, Nov. 25, 1992.

McAuliffe, Kathleen. "Interview: W. French Anderson." *Omni*, July 1991.

Mann, Jonathan M., et al. "The International Epidemiology of AIDS." *Scientific American*, Oct. 1988.

Marrack, Philippa, and John Kappler. "The T Cell and Its Receptor." *Scientific American*, Feb. 1986.

Marx, Jean. "Taming Rogue Immune Reactions." *Science*, July 20, 1990.

Matthews, Thomas J., and Dani P. Bolognesi. "AIDS Vaccines." *Scientific American*, Oct. 1988.

"New Weapons to Defend the Body against Itself." *Business Week*, Dec. 3, 1990.

Nowak, Rachel. "Diversity Equals Death." *Discover*, May 1992.

Old, Lloyd J. "Tumor Necrosis Factor." *Scientific American*, May 1988.

Ota, Kohei, et al. "T-Cell Recognition of an Immunodominant Myelin Basic Protein Epitope in Multiple Sclerosis." *Nature*, July 12, 1990.

Palca, Joseph. "Testing Target Date Looms, but Will the Vaccines Be Ready?" *Science*, Sept. 11, 1992.

Paliard, Xavier, et al. "Evidence for the Effects of a Superantigen in Rheumatoid Arthritis." *Science*, July 19, 1991.

Patlak, Margie. "The Arsenal Gets Larger." *Discover*, Apr. 1989.

Pennisi, E. "Cancer Cells Caught in the (Metastatic) Act." *Science News*, May 22, 1993.

Redfield, Robert R., and Donald S. Burke. "HIV Infection: The Clinical Picture." *Scientific American*, Oct. 1988.

Rennie, John:
"The Body against Itself." *Scientific American*, Dec. 1990.
"Keeping It in the Family." *Scientific American*, Aug. 1992.

Rosenberg, Steven A. "Adoptive Immunotherapy for Cancer." *Scientific American*, May 1990.

Russell, Cristine. "Louis Pasteur and Questions of Fraud." *Washington Post*, Feb. 23, 1993.

Sharma, Hari M., Brihaspati Dev Triguna, and Deepak Chopra. "Maharishi Ayur-Veda: Modern Insights into Ancient Medicine." JAMA, May 22/29, 1991.

Silberner, Joanne. "Chipping Away at AIDS." *U.S. News & World Report*, Apr. 9, 1990.

Sinha, Animesh A., M. Theresa Lopez, and Hugh O. McDevitt. "Autoimmune Diseases: The Failure of Self Tolerance." *Science*, June 15, 1990.

"Some Progress Is Reported in Test of Gene Therapy." *New York Times*, Feb. 19, 1991.

"Testing of Autoimmune Therapy Begins." *Science*, Apr. 5, 1991.

Todd, John. "A Most Intimate Foe." *The Sciences*, Mar./Apr. 1990.

Tonegawa, Susumu. "The Molecules of the Immune System." *Scientific American*, Oct. 1985.

Toufexis, Anastasia. "Dr. Jacob's Alternative Mission." *Time*, Mar. 1, 1993.

Ungeheuer, Frederick. "The Master Detective, Still on the Case." *Time*, Aug. 3, 1992.

Valentine, Martin D. "Anaphylaxis and Stinging Insect Hypersensitivity." JAMA, Nov. 25, 1992.

Verma, Inder M. "Gene Therapy." *Scientific American*, Nov. 1990.

"Virus on the Run." U.S. *News & World Report*, Nov. 19, 1990.

Weaver, Robert F. "Beyond Supermouse: Changing Life's Genetic Blueprint." *National Geographic*, Dec. 1984.

Weber, Jonathan N., and Robin A. Weiss. "HIV Infection: The Cellular Picture." *Scientific American*, Oct. 1988.

Wechsler, Rob. "A New Prescription: Mind over Malady." *Discover*, Feb. 1987.

Weisse, Allen B. "Of Birds and Blood Cells." *Hospital Practice*, July 15, 1992.

Winter, Greg, and William J. Harris. "Humanized Antibodies." *Immunology Today*, June 1993.

Yarchoan, Robert, Hiroaki Mitsuya, and Samuel Broder. "AIDS Therapies." *Scientific American*, Oct. 1988.

Young, John Ding-E, and Zanvil A. Cohn. "How Killer Cells Kill." *Scientific American*, Jan. 1988.

OTHER SOURCES:

Budd, Matthew A. "Human Suffering: The Road to Illness or the Gateway to Learning." Lecture at conference. Lee Travis Institute for Biopsychosocial Research and the U.S. Public Health Service, Nov. 13, 1992.

"Horizons of Cancer Research: Progress and Prospects." National Cancer Institute, NIH Publication No. 89-3011. Bethesda, Md.: National Institutes of Health, Dec. 1988.

Schindler, Lydia Woods:
"The Immune System—How It Works." NIH Publication No. 92-3229. Bethesda, Md.: National Institutes of Health, June 1992.
"Understanding the Immune System." Revised. NIH Publication No. 92-529. Bethesda, Md.: National Institutes of Health, Oct. 1991.

INDEX

Page numbers in boldface refer to illustrations or illustrated text.

A

Acquired immunity, 38-60, 61, **64-65, 66-67, 68-69;** ancient understanding of, 43; antiantibodies, 56, 58; antibiotics, effect of, **59-60;** chemical network in, 55-56; Ehrlich's theory, 50-51; inflammatory response, **48-49,** 66; Koch, work of, 43-44; Pasteur, work of, 43-44, 46-47; polio vaccines, 58-59; B cell receptors' role in, **42;** to smallpox, 38, 40-**41,** 43. *See also* Antibodies; B cells; T cells

Acquired immunodeficiency syndrome (AIDS), 73, 84, 86-93, **90-91**

Activation of immune cell, defined, 64

Adenosine deaminase (ADA) deficiency, 84

Ader, Robert, 105-106, **107**

Adrenal glands, cortisol released by, **116**

AIDS (acquired immunodeficiency syndrome), 73, 84, 86-93, **90-91**

Allergies, **94-99;** asthma as, 95, 106; causes, **94-95;** histamine release, **50-51,** 58, **97;** multiple chemical sensitivities (MCS), 85; process, **96-97;** treatment, 58, **98-99;** types, 99

Allison, Bobby, **118**

Allison, V. D., 22

Amino acid chains, receptors as, **42**

Amoeba, **12**

Anandamide, 113; receptors, **112-113**

Anthrax bacteria, 20, 44, 46

Antiantibodies, concept of, 56, 58, 99

Antibiotics, effect of, **59**-60

Antibodies, 21, 43, 52-54; in allergic reactions, 58, **96-97**; in allergy treatment, **98-99**; in autoimmunity treatment, 82; on B cell surface, **65**; cancer cells and, **128**; in cancer therapy, **130-131**; and complement, 21, **48, 49,** 66; in Ehrlich's theory, 50; to HIV, 90, 91; in lupus, 72, **73,** 76; from plasma cells, 44, 53-54, **65, 66, 68, 86, 96, 98, 130-131**; receptors and, 42; rheumatoid factors, 79

Antigens, 53; allergens, **94-95, 96, 97, 98-99;** amoeba, **12;** cancer cells', 124, **128;** and complement, 21, **48, 49,** 66; epitopes, **42;** in lymphatic system, 36, 37; MHC and, 28, **63, 64-65,** 80; parasites, **15, 52-53;** superantigens, 77, **78,** 79; T cells' reactions, learning of, 35. *See also* Bacteria; Viruses

Antitoxin, discovery of, 21, 50

Arthritis, rheumatoid: effects, **70-71,** 77, 79, **81;** emotional factors in, 105; treatments, possible, 81, 82

Asthma, conditioning of, 106

Autoimmune diseases, 60, 70-82; AIDS as, 73, 90-91; autoreactive cells in, 74-75, 76, 77, 80; genetics and, 79-80, 82; lupus, 9-10, 70, 72, **73,** 76-77, 106; molecular-mimicry theory, 75-76; multiple sclerosis (MS), 74-75, **76;** rheumatoid arthritis (RA), **70-71,** 77, 79, **81,** 105; sex hormones and, 76-77; skepticism about, 72; superantigens and, 77, **78,** 79; treatments, possible, 81-82

Autoreactive (autoimmune) cells, **70-71, 73,** 74-75, 76, 77, 80

Azidothymidine (AZT), 91-92

B

Bacteria: antibiotic's effect on, **59;** blood serum as killer of, 20; friendly vs. unfriendly, 22, 24; inflammatory response to, **48-49;** Koch's work with, 44; lysozyme as killer of, 22, 25; macrophage and, **8-9;** Pasteur's work with, 44, 46; streptococcal, **13,** 75

Bartók, Béla, 100

Basophils, 96-97

B cells, **36, 37,** 54, **55,** 64, **65;** in allergy, **96, 98, 99;** IL-2 and, 56; and lupus victims' antibodies, 72, **73,** 76; memory, **49, 65, 68,** 69, **96;** receptors, **42, 65.** *See also* Plasma cells

Behavioral Immunology Committee, National Institutes of Health, 122

Behring, Emil von, 20-21, 50

Belokopitova, Olga, 14, 15

Besedovsky, Hugo, work of, 106-107

Billingham, Rupert, 26

Biofeedback for relaxation, 120, **122**

Biologicals in cancer therapy, **130-131**

Blalock, Edwin, 108

Blood cells. *See* Red blood cells; White blood cells

Blood serum, role of, 20, 21

Bolognesi, Dani, 91

Bone marrow, **32-33, 56-57;** transplants, 83

Bordet, Jules, 21, 51

Brain: HIV and, 88; immune system links with, 106-108, **112-113,** 115, **116-117,** 120; in multiple sclerosis, **76;** receptors, 107-108, **112**

Breast cancer, mental state and, 102

Brent, Leslie, 26

Bubble Boy (David; SCID patient), 82-84, **83**

Bubonic plague, Procopius's account of, 43

Budd, Matthew, 111

Bulloch, Karen, 107

Burnet, Macfarlane, 25, 26; clonal selection theory, 53-54

Buying the pox (ingrafting), 40

C

Cancer, **124-133;** in AIDS patients, 86; breast, mental state and, 102; holistic approaches, 104, 114, 121; immune system evaded by, **128-129;** killer cells vs., **125, 127, 130-131, 132-133;** metastasis, 119, 124, **127;** new therapies, **130-131;** placebo response in, 103-104; Type C coping and, 115, 118-119

Candida albicans (yeast), spores of, **19**

Capillaries, 36; in inflammation, **48-49;** sinusoidal, **32-33**

Cell-mediated vs. humoral response, 66

Cellular vs. humoral theorists, 20, 50, 51

Cholera, Pasteur's study of, 44, 46

Cilia: sperm and, **28-29;** in trachea, **16-17, 62-63,** 89

Clonal selection theory, 53-54

Cognitive therapy, 111-112, 114

Complement proteins, **21;** and inflammation, **48, 49,** 66

Conditioned responses, 105-106

Contact hypersensitivities, 99

Coping style and cancer, 115, 118-119

Cortisol, release of, **116**

Cousins, Norman, 100

Cowpox, immunity to smallpox conferred by, 38, 40-**41,** 43

Cytokines: interferon, 25, 56, 63, 130; IL-1, 81, 115; IL-2, 56, 84, **130-131;** macrophages' release of, **63, 64, 96;** T cells' release of, **64-65, 96, 99;** therapies blocking, 81-82

Cytotoxic T cells. *See* Killer T cells

D

Dander as allergen, **94**

David the Bubble Boy (SCID patient), 82-84, **83**

Davis, Mark, quoted, 55

Del Rey, Adriana, work of, 106-107

DeSilva, Ashanthi, 84

Devane, William, 113

Diabetes, juvenile, genetics and, 79-80

DNA (deoxyribonucleic acid): in autoimmunity, 72; and cancer, **126;** virus's, **14**

E

E. *coli* bacteria, macrophage and, **8-9**

Ehrlich, Paul, 50-51, 56, 58, 72

Embryos, development of, 26, 30

Emotions. *See* Psychoneuroimmunology

Endorphins, 108; in Type C coping, 118

Epinephrine, action of, **117**

Epitopes, receptors and, **42**

Experimental allergic encephalomyelitis (EAE), 74, 82

F

Felten, David, 107, **110**, 123
Fibrin, tumor encapsulated in, **129**
Fight-or-flight response, 109, 115, **116-117**
Fleming, Alexander, 22, **24**
Friendly flora, **19**, 22, 24

G

Galen (Greek physician), 102
Gallo, Robert, 87
Genetics: of allergies, 95; of autoimmunity, 79-80, 82; of B cell receptors, 42; of cancer, **126**; of histocompatibility types, 26, 80; of immunodeficiencies, 84
Germ theory of disease, 13
Gibson, Thomas, 25
Goblet cells, cilia and, in trachea, **16-17**
Gowans, James L., 54
Graaf, Reinier de, 12
Graft-rejection process, 25-26
Graft versus host disease (GVHD), 83

H

Haase, Ashley, 75
Hafler, David, 74
Hairs, **16**
Hall, Nick, 121
Hand, rheumatoid arthritis in, **70-71**
Hay fever, causes of, **94-95**
Helper T cells, **55**, 56, 64, **65**; in allergy, **96**, **98**, **99**; cancer and, **129**; HIV and, 88-89; superantigens' stimulation of, **78**, 79
Hindu practices: inoculation, ancient, 43; oil treatment, **121**
Hiserodt, John, quoted, 119
Histamine, **50-51**, 58, 66. See also Mediators of inflammation
Histocompatibility types, 26, 80
HIV (human immunodeficiency virus), 73, 87-89, **90-91**, 92-93
HLA-DQ (gene), 80
Hoffmann, Geoffrey, theory by, 90-91
Holistic healthcare, 104; cognitive therapy, 111-112, 114; relaxation techniques, 119-

121, **122**
Hooke, Robert, 13
Hormones: cortisol, release of, **116**; immune system's manufacture of, 108; in reaction to superantigens, **78**, 79; sex hormones and lupus, 76-77
HTLV-1, -2, and -3 (viruses), 87
Hughes, Josephine, **85**
Human immunodeficiency virus (HIV), 73, 87-89, **90-91**, 92-93
Human T-cell lymphotropic viruses, 87
Humoral immunity, 21; vs. cellular theory, 20, 50, 51
Humoral vs. cell-mediated response, 66
Hypersensitivities. See Allergies
Hypnosis for relaxation, 120, **122**
Hypothalamus and immune system suppression, 115, **116-117**

I

Imagery, mental, 104, 120-121
Immune system, 10-11; example of response, **61-69**; history of study, **10-11**, 12-15, 20-22, **24**, 50-51; immunodeficiencies, 73, 82-84, **83**, 86-93, **90-91**; skin, 11, **16**, **18-19**, 25, 26; sperm and, **28-29**, 30. See also Acquired immunity; Allergies; Antibodies; Antigens; Autoimmune diseases; Cancer; Lymphatic system; MHC; Psychoneuroimmunology
Immunodeficiency diseases, 73, 82-84; AIDS, 73, 84, 86-93, **90-91**; SCID, cases of, 82-84, **83**; secondary, kinds of, 84
Immunoglobulins (Ig), 53, 54; allergies and, 58, **96-97**, **98-99**; in lupus, 72
Inflammation, **48-49**, 66; mediators of, **97**; in rheumatoid arthritis, 77, 79, 81
Influenza, immune response in, **61-69**
Ingrafting (buying the pox), 40
Innate immune response, 61, **62-63**
Inoculation: ancient form of, 43. See also Vaccinations
Insulin insufficiency in diabetes, 80
Interferon, 25, 56, 63, 130
Interleukin-1 (IL-1), 81, 115
Interleukin-2 (IL-2), 56, 84; in cancer therapy, **130-131**

Interstitial fluid, 37
Intestinal tract, mucus in, **19**
Isaacs, Alick, 25

J

Jenner, Edward, 38, 40-**41**
Jerne, Niels Kaj, 58
Jesty, Benjamin, 40
Juvenile diabetes, genetics and, 79-80

K

Kaposi's sarcoma, 86
Kappler, John, 77, 79
Kidney disease, lupus as, 70, 72
Killer T cells, 55, **64**, **66-67**; vs. cancer, **129**, **130-131**, **132-133**; vs. HIV, 87; MHC system and, 26, 28
Kirkpatrick, Richard, case report by, 9-10
Kitasato, Shibasaburo, 50
Koch, Robert, 13, 43-44, 50
Krebiozen (drug) as placebo, 103-104

L

Landsteiner, Karl, 52
LAV (lymphadenopathy-associated virus), 87
Learned helplessness, 111
Leeuwenhoek, Antoni van, 12-13
Leonard, Michael, 93
Leukocytes. See White blood cells
Levy, Sandra, 111, 114
Limbic system: anandamide receptors in, **112**; relaxation and, 120
Lindenmann, Jean, 25
Liver cells in lupus, **73**
Lourdes, France, cures at, 102
Lungs, particles inhaled into, **88-89**
Lupus, 70, 72, 76-77; and conditioning, 106; liver in, **73**; and witchcraft, 9-10
Lymph, 36, 37
Lymphadenopathy-associated virus (LAV), 87
Lymphatic system, **31-37**; bone marrow, **32-33**, **56-57**, 83; lymph nodes, **36**, **47**; metastasis and, 127; nerve pathways to, 107, **110**, **117**; spleen, 37, 107, **110**, **113**; thymus, **34-35**, 54-55, 74, **117**

Lymphatic vessels, **36-37**

Lymph nodes, **36**, **47**

Lymphocytes, 20, 32, 33, 54, **125**; natural killer cells, 55, 119, **127**; vaccination and, 43. *See also* B cells; T cells

Lymphokine, IL-2 as, 56, 84, **130-131**

Lysozyme, 22, 25

M

Macaulay, Thomas, quoted, 40

McDevitt, Hugh, 80

McGregor, Douglas, 54

Macrophages, 15, 23, 56; allergens and, **96**, 99; and bacteria, **8-9**, 23; and cancer cells, **127**, **129**; cleanup, **69**; epinephrine and, **117**; helper T cells and, **64-65**, **96**, **98**; HIV in, 88; IL-1 from, 115; and inhaled particles, **88-89**; and neuropeptides, 108; and red blood cell, **23**; and viruses, **62-63**

Major histocompatibility complex. *See* MHC

Malaria organisms, action of, **52-53**

Marrack, Philippa, 77, 79

Marrow, **32-33**, **56-57**; transplants, 83

Massage for relaxation, **121**

Mast cells, 96-**97**, **98-99**

Measles and multiple sclerosis, 75

Medawar, Peter, 25-26

Mediators of inflammation, **97**

Meditation for relaxation, 120

Memory cells, 54, 56, **64**, **65**, **68**, 69, 131; in allergy, **96**; in inflammation, **48**

Mental imagery, 104, 120-121

Metastasis of cancer, 119, 124, **127**

Metchnikoff, Élie, **10-11**, 14-15, 20, 50

MHC (major histocompatibility complex), 26, **27**, 28, 54; antigens and, **63**, **64-65**, **78**, 79, **96**; and HIV, 90, 91; and juvenile diabetes, 80; T cells' reactions, learning of, 35

Miasma vs. germ theories of disease, 13

Microscope, history of, 12-13

Miller, Jacques, 54

Mind-body link. *See* Psychoneuroimmu-nology

Molecular mimicry, theory of, 75-76

Montagnier, Luc, 87, 90

MRI brain scan in multiple sclerosis, **76**

Mucous membranes, **16-17**; sperm and, **28-29**

Mucus, **19**; lysozyme in, 22

Multiple chemical sensitivities (MCS), 85

Multiple sclerosis (MS), 74-75; brain in, **76**; treatments, possible, 82

Myelin destruction in multiple sclerosis, 74-75, **76**

N

Natural killer (NK) cells, 55; cancer and, 119, **127**; massage for enhancing, **121**

Nelmes, Sarah, 40

Nepom, Gerald, 80

Nerve cells: AIDS and, 88; immune system, pathways to, 107, **110**, **117**; multiple sclerosis damage, 74, **76**; synapse, **109**

Network theory of antiantibodies, 58

Neuropeptides, 108

Neurotransmitters: anandamide, receptors for, **112-113**; epinephrine, action of, **117**; synaptic vesicles for, **109**

Neutrophils, **48**, **49**; killed by cancer, **129**

Nonspecific immune response, **62-63**

Nuttall, George, 20

O

Office of Alternative Medicine (OAM), National Institutes of Health, 122

Oil treatment for relaxation, **121**

Olness, Karen, 106

Oncogenes, action of, **126**

Opiate receptors, brain's, 107-108

Optimism vs. pessimism, 109-112, 114

Owen, Ray, 26

P

Pancreas in juvenile diabetes, 80

Parasites, **15**; malaria, **52-53**

Passive immunity, 54

Pasteur, Louis, 13, 43-44, 46-47

Pauling, Linus, 52-53

Pavlov, Ivan, 105

Penicillin, 59-60; as allergen, **94-95**

Peptides: MHC molecule with, **27**; neuropeptides, 108

Perforins, release of, 66, **67**

Pert, Candace, 107-108, 123

Pessimism vs. optimism, 109-112, 114

Peterson, Christopher, 110, 111

Phagocytes, 15, 20, **23**, 51; Metchnikoff and, 11, 15, 20; neutrophils, **48**, **49**, **129**. *See also* Macrophages

Phipps, James, 40, **41**

Placebo response, 102-104, 105

Plaques in multiple sclerosis, 74, **76**

Plasma, 36-37

Plasma cells, 36, **44-45**, **65**, **66**, **68**; allergens and, **96**, **98**; in clonal selection theory, 53-54; in experimental therapies, **86**, **130-131**

Platelets, **38-39**

Polio vaccines, 58-59

Pollen as allergen, 58, **94-95**

Pre-T cells, maturing in thymus, **34-35**

Procopius (Byzantine historian), quoted, 43

Proto-oncogenes, **126**

Pseudopods, macrophages', **8-9**, 62

Psychoneuroimmunology (PNI), 100-123; and AIDS, 93; and allergies, 95; brain's links with immune system, 106-108, **112-113**, 115, **116-117**, 120; conditioned responses, 105-106; emotional expression, 114, **118**; future of, 122-123; and metastasis, 119; nerve pathways to immune system, 107, **110**, **117**; pessimism vs. optimism, 109-112, 114; placebo response, 102-104, 105; relaxation techniques, 119-**121**, **122**; and rheumatoid arthritis, 105; stress effects, 109, 114, 115, **116-117**; Type C behavior, 115, 118-119; witchcraft, case of, 9-10

Pus: phagocytes in, 15; smallpox treatment with, 40, **41**

R

Rabies, Pasteur's work with, 46-47
Ragweed allergy treatment, possible, 58
Receptors: anandamide, **112-113;** B cells', **42;** Burnet's theory, 53; Ehrlich's side chains, 50; IL-2, lack of, 84; macro-phage's, **117;** neuropeptide, 108; opiate, 107-108; T cells', 35, 77, **116**
Red blood cells, **38-39;** amoeba's inges-tion of, 12; in bone marrow, **56-57;** in inflammation, **48, 49;** and macrophages, **8-9, 23;** in malaria infection, **52-53**
Red marrow, **32-33, 56-57;** transplants, 83
Red pulp in spleen, **37**
Rejection of tissue, 25-26
Relaxation techniques, 119-**121, 122**
Renoux, Gerard, 107
Repressor (Type C) personality, 115, 118-119
Reproductive tract: sperm, **28-29,** 30; yeast, **19**
Respiratory tract: asthma, 106; bacteria at-tacking, **13;** cilia in, **16-17;** inhaled parti-cles in, **88-89;** virus attacking, **14**
Rheumatic fever, 75
Rheumatoid arthritis (RA): effects of, **70-71,** 77, 79, **81;** emotional factors in, 105; treatments, possible, 81, 82
Rheumatoid (R) factors, 79
Ruff, Michael, 108

S

Sabin, Albert, 58
Salk, Jonas, 58, 92, 123
Scalp: hairs, **16;** skin flakes from, **18-19**
Schan, Wendy, 121
Schistosome, **15**
SCID (severe combined immunodeficiency), 73; cases of, 82-84, **83**
Self vs. other, concept of, 10-11, 26, 61, 99; in cancer, 124, **128.** *See also* MHC
Seligman, Martin, 111, 112, 114, 119, 123
Serum, blood, role of, 20, 21
Severe combined immunodeficiency

(SCID), 73; cases of, 82-84, **83**
Sex hormones and lupus, 76-77
Shenk, Marsha, 100
Shirodhara drip for relaxation, **121**
Side chains in Ehrlich's theory, 50
Simonton, Carl and Stephanie, 104
Skeletal structure of body, **33**
Skin: breaks in, and inflammatory re-sponse, **48-49;** as first line of defense, 11, **16, 18-19;** grafts, 25, 26
Smallpox, 38, 40; prevention, 40-**41,** 43
Smith, Kendall A., 56
Snyder, Solomon, 107
Solomon, George, 105
Somatizers, 114
Sorkin, Ernst, work of, 106-107
Specific immunity. *See* Acquired immunity
Sperm cells, **28-29,** 30
Spleen, **37;** anandamide receptors, **113;** nerve pathways to, 107, **110**
Staphylococci, antibiotics' effect on, **59**
Stem cells, 32
Stott, E. J., 91
Streptococci, **13;** and rheumatic fever, 75
Stress and immune system, 109, 115, **116-117;** relieving, means of, 119-**121, 122;** somatization, 114; witchcraft case, 10
Strominger, Jack, 28
Superantigens, 77, **78,** 79
Suppressor T cells, 55, **99**
Sweat, **18**
Synapse and synaptic vesicles, **109**

T

T cells, **36-37;** in autoimmunity, 74-75, 77, 79, 80; cortisol in, **116;** in gene thera-py, 84; HIV and, 87, 88-89, 90; in lymph nodes, 36; maturation of, in thymus, **34-35,** 54-55; memory, **64, 68,** 69; superanti-gens and, 77, **78,** 79; suppressor, 55, **99;** types of, 55. *See also* Helper T cells; Killer T cells
Tears, lysozyme in, 22
Temoshok, Lydia, 115, 118, 119

Template theory of antibody formation, 53
Tetrahydrocannabinol (THC), 113
Thighbone, rheumatoid arthritis in, **81**
Thucydides (Greek historian), quoted, 43
Thymus, **34-35,** 54-55, 74; nerve signals to, **117**
Tissue rejection and compatibility, 25-26
Trachea: cilia, **16-17,** 89; influenza in, **61-69**
Tumors. *See* Cancer
Type A vs. Type B people, 115
Type C behavior, 115, 118-119

V

Vaccinations, 54, 69; AIDS, possible, 91, 92; autoimmune disease, 82; Pasteur, work of, 44, 46-47; polio, 58-59; smallpox, de-velopment of, 38, 40-**41,** 43
Vernier, Robert, 70, 72
Viruses, **14,** 24-25, 60; formation of, **62;** HIV, 73, 87-89, **90-91,** 92-93; influenza, im-mune response to, **61-69;** vs. interferon, 25, 56, 63; vs. killer T cells, 55; measles, and multiple sclerosis, 75; in polio vac-cine, 58-59; rabies, 46-47; smallpox, fight against, 38, 40-**41,** 43
Visintainer, Madelon, 119
Visualization technique, 104, 120-121
Vittini, Jackie, **103**

W

Webeck, Ron, 93
Weiner, Howard, 74
White blood cells, 31, **38-39;** basophils, 96-97; bone marrow as source of, **32-33, 56-57;** Ehrlich's theory, 50-51; neutro-phils, **48, 49, 129.** *See also* Lymphocytes; Phagocytes
White pulp in spleen, **37**
Witch doctor, lupus case treated by, 9-10
Wonder drugs, effect of, **59-60**

Y

Yeast spores, **19**

ACKNOWLEDGMENTS

The editors of *Defending Army* would like to thank these individuals for their valuable contributions:

Julia Albright, George Washington University, Washington, D.C.; Mel Auston, Bethesda, Maryland; Jim Benjamin, Millersville, Maryland; Matthew Budd, Harvard Community Health Plan, Boston; Mark H. Ellisman, University of California, San Diego; David Felten, University of Rochester, Rochester, New York; Constance Garnett, Harvard University, Cambridge, Massachusetts; David Hafler, Brigham and Women's Hospital, Boston; Miles Herkenham, National Institutes of Health, Bethesda, Maryland; Richard Kirkpatrick, Longview, Washington; Dean Madden, Max-Planck-Institut für Medizinische Forschung, Heidelberg; Don Monroe, Howard University, Washington, D.C.; Terry Moody, George Washington University, Washington, D.C.; Candace Pert, Peptide Research, Rockville, Maryland; Julia Roland, Georgetown University, Washington, D.C.; Michael Ruff, Peptide Research, Rockville, Maryland; Wendy Schan, Long Beach Memorial Center, Long Beach, California; Marsha Shenk, Napa, California; Elizabeth T. Stout, Harvard Community Health Plan, Boston; Lydia Temoshok, Henry M. Jackson Foundation for Advancement of Military Medicine, Rockville, Maryland; Robert Vernier, University of Minnesota, Minneapolis; Don Wiley, Harvard University, Cambridge, Massachusetts.

PICTURE CREDITS